Communication Skills for Mental Health Nurses

Jean Morrissey
Patrick Callaghan

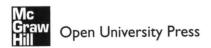
Open University Press

Open University Press
McGraw-Hill Education
McGraw-Hill House
Shoppenhangers Road
Maidenhead
Berkshire
England
SL6 2QL

email: enquiries@openup.co.uk
world wide web: www.openup.co.uk

and Two Penn Plaza, New York, NY 10121-2289, USA

First published 2011

A catalogue record of this book is available from the British Library

ISBN-13: 978-0-33-523870-5 (pb) 978-0-33-523871-2 (hb)
ISBN-10: 033523870X (pb) 0335238718 (hb)
e-ISBN: 9780335238729

Library of Congress Cataloging-in-Publication Data
CIP data applied for

Typeset by Aptara Inc., India
Printed in the UK by Bell and Bain Ltd, Glasgow

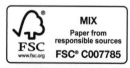

MIX
Paper from
responsible sources
FSC
www.fsc.org FSC® C007785

The McGraw·Hill Companies

Contents

About the Authors

Jean Morrissey is a lecturer in mental health nursing at the School of Nursing, Trinity College Dublin. She is also an accredited counsellor and clinical supervisor. She has worked for many years as a mental health nurse in hospital and community settings, and as a nurse educator in various educational settings in the UK and Hong Kong. Her research interests include communication and counselling, suicidality and self-harm, clinical supervision and working with diversity and mental health care. She is currently reading for a PhD at Trinity College Dublin.

Patrick Callaghan is Professor of Mental Health Nursing and Director of Research at the School of Nursing, Midwifery and Physiotherapy at the University of Nottingham where he leads the Mental Health Research Programme. He is Visiting Professor in Mental Health at Trinity College Dublin and a Professorial Fellow of the Institute of Mental Health, Nottingham. He is a Chartered Health Psychologist and Chartered Health Scientist and has worked in mental health for 26 years. His research interests are evaluating psychosocial interventions, testing social cognition models of health-related behaviour and mental health nursing policy and service evaluation.

Acknowledgements

We appreciate and value the knowledge, experience and learning gained from all the clients/service users, family members and carers, students and colleagues with whom we have worked with over the years.

Preface

There is no doubt that communication in mental health nursing is a fundamental component of all therapeutic interventions. The knowledge and interpersonal skills that a mental health nurse uses to communicate are important aspects of helping the person who is experiencing mental health problems as well as facilitating the development of a positive nurse–service user relationship. As such we believe that this requires nurses to demonstrate a range of appropriate and effective communication and engagement skills with individuals who have mental health problems, their carers and other key people involved in their care. In 1952, Hildegard Peplau, an American psychiatric nurse, wrote a seminal work on interpersonal relations in nursing. In her book, Peplau argued that effective communication skills were central to sound interpersonal skills and fundamental to the role of mental health nurses. Over 50 years later, this view remains central to the work of mental health nurses. Mental health nursing is essentially a professional helping relationship in which nurses have a responsibility to be person-centred, self-aware, reflect on their ability to analyse their own feelings, model effective interpersonal skills to others, act selflessly and ethically, and be tolerant, empathetic, sensitive, trustworthy, caring and friendly.

The aim of this book is to introduce students embarking on a career in mental health nursing to key aspects of communication theory and practice, and help equip them with the knowledge and skills to develop and hone effective communication in clinical practice. Our aim in producing this book was to make it as comprehensive as possible, but inevitably constraints of space meant that we had to omit areas we might ideally have liked to have included. Accordingly, we decided to include the areas that we believe are of most importance both to novice nurses and indeed more experienced practitioners seeking to update their knowledge in specific areas of communication. This book will be a practical guide to those communication skills and interventions needed by nurses who are participating in high-quality nursing care for people with a variety of mental health problems in different clinical settings. Throughout this book emphasis is placed in each chapter on the application of communication skills and interventions, which are illustrated through the use of clinical examples. The importance of applying theory to practice is paramount and this theme is illustrated by clinical case studies. Each chapter concludes with reflective questions designed to help readers consolidate their learning from the book and point them in the direction of further learning on the subject.

The book comprises 11 chapters and begins with an introduction to the core communication skills that are most relevant to mental health nursing and their application to practice. Chapter 2 addresses the values, culture and evidence-based communication styles designed to foster recovery in people living with mental distress and promote their sense of wellbeing through the adoption of positive mental health nursing. Chapter 3 examines the concept of reflection and its usefulness in enhancing nurses' learning, as well as its value in developing the skills required for effective communication. This is followed by the use and value of phatic communication, and brief ordinary and effective communication in mental health nursing. Chapter 5 presents Heron's (2001) Six Category Intervention Analysis model of communication and its application in mental health practice. The next four chapters focus on issues relating to communicating across cultures, professional helping relationships, assertive communication and resolving conflict in mental health practice. The final two chapters present two communication approaches, namely solution-focused interventions and motivational interviewing, and their clinical application.

Finally, we hope that this book will inform and inspire the reader and act as a springboard for ongoing reflection, discussion, practice and learning concerning the knowledge and use of appropriate and effective communication and engagement skills that a mental health nurse applies to communicate with individuals who have mental health problems, their carers and other key people involved in their care within an ever-changing therapeutic environment.

Jean Morrissey and Patrick Callaghan

Core communication skills in mental health nursing

Introduction

Communication in mental health nursing is an essential component of all therapeutic interventions. The knowledge and interpersonal skills that a nurse uses to communicate are essential aspects of helping the person who is experiencing mental health problems or distress, as well as facilitating the development of a positive nurse–client relationship. This requires the mental health nurse to use a range of appropriate and effective communication and engagement skills with individuals, their carers and other significant people involved in their care. This chapter examines the verbal and non-verbal communication skills that are most relevant to mental health nursing, and illustrates how each skill can be used in practice.

Learning outcomes

By the end of this chapter, you should be better able to:

1 describe the components of therapeutic communication skills
2 demonstrate an understanding of how the different communication skills can be used in clinical practice
3 use interpersonal skills in clinical practice.

Interpersonal skills

Effective interpersonal skills are central to a mental health nurse's ability to form a sound therapeutic alliance and to the role of mental health nurses (Peplau, 1952). In mental health nursing, communication skills form the basis of every intervention. Good interpersonal skills are what each mental health nurse needs to make nursing happen. These skills are the building blocks or, as Stevenson (2008, p.109) describes them, 'the nuts and bolts – the basic techniques and principles in which everyone engaging in clinical practice in mental health needs to be fluent'. In order to communicate effectively the mental health nurse needs to work towards being proficient in using the basic communication tools; this means knowing what skill s/he is using and why, and being able to move skilfully from one skill to another as and when the purpose of the interaction requires. In addition, given that different clients have different needs, it is inevitable that mental health nurses will use different skills with different clients in various mental health settings. As Stevenson (2008, p.109) points out, 'one size does not fit all'.

Interpersonal skills that are commonly used in mental health practice are described below. Each skill is explained and supported with specific examples and exercises. These descriptions are by no means intended to be exhaustive or prescriptive but instead we aim to provide the general principles for the use of each skill presented. Each skill is described as a stand-alone piece of communication; however, it is important to remember that when used in practice, these skills will be used interdependently. Furthermore, 'when all the skills are being used together, the mental health nurse provides the proper, respectful conditions that facilitate a positive change to occur' (Stickley and Stacey, 2009, p.47). The following communication skills will be explained:

- listening
- paraphrasing
- summarizing
- questioning
- non-verbal communication.

Listening

Listening is the most important skill and often the most challenging. In our experience, mental health nurses often worry about what they are going to say, what questions they should ask, or whether they have asked the *right* question. While such concerns are common and understandable for the newcomer to mental health nursing, these thoughts can distract the mental health nurse from listening to the person who is talking. One of the common mistakes made by novice mental health nurses as well as experienced nurses is to talk too much. When we are talking, we are not listening! The best and the most therapeutic thing to do is to say less and listen more. Mental health nurses and indeed other helping practitioners, however, often find this difficult. One common reason for this is that many mental health nurses believe they are not doing anything when they are *just* listening (Bonham, 2004) and as a result they underestimate the value of simply listening and more importantly its therapeutic effect. Listening to a client does not mean that you are doing nothing; instead, you are allowing a space for the person to talk. Stevenson (2008, p.110) echoes this and states that 'even if the mental health nurse does nothing but listen, there is likely to be a therapeutic effect'. Several studies have also reported that people who used mental health services value having the opportunity to tell their story and more importantly being heard (Jensen, 2000; Kai and Crosland, 2001; Moyle, 2003; Koivisto et al., 2004; Gilburt et al., 2008; Hopkins et al., 2009).

Listening helps clients to:

- feel cared about and accepted
- feel significant and respected
- feel heard and understood
- connect with other people
- establish a sense of trust with helper(s)
- feel less isolated and alone
- make sense of their current situations and/or past experiences
- ask for help
- give feedback about their care
- express emotions and release tensions
- participate in their care planning.

Listening is clearly an essential component of effective communication as well as being one of the most important interventions the mental health nurse can offer to a service user. However, listening means more than just hearing the words spoken by the person, it involves *active* listening (McCabe and Timmins, 2006). Listening actively means giving your full attention – that is physically, mentally and emotionally – which needs to be communicated to the person who is talking. Effective listening is therefore a cognitive, behavioural and an affective process (Arnold and Underman Boggs, 2003). Developing a capacity to listen, and trying to understand the client's experience is a challenge for the novice mental health nurse. Similar to acquiring any new skill, learning how to listen effectively takes time and plenty of practice.

Listening involves the following:

- providing time for the person to tell his/her story
- offering a quiet and private space, free from distractions to listen to the person
- listening with the purpose of understanding the person's message
- giving full attention by focusing on what the person is saying
- tuning out external distractions, such as background noises
- tuning out internal distractions, such as thoughts about what to say next.

Listening skills involve using a range of verbal and non-verbal continuation prompts – for example, verbal prompts include:

- 'Mmm' 'Yes'
- 'Absolutely' 'I see'
- 'Please continue' 'Oh'
- 'Say more about' 'Really'
- 'Go on' 'So'.

Non-verbal behaviours include:

- showing it in your face, for example facial expression, looking interested and concerned; maintaining good eye contact

- showing it in your body movements, for example nodding of head, leaning forward.

Listening to non-verbal communication

Much of the communication that takes place between people is non-verbal. Our faces and bodies are extremely communicative. Being able to read non-verbal messages or body language is an important factor in establishing and maintaining relationships (Carton et al., 1999).

Body language includes many different aspects of non-verbal behaviour, including:

- eye contact such as staring, avoiding eye contact
- facial expressions such as frowning, smiling, clenching or 'biting' lips, raising eyebrows
- voice, such as tone, volume, accent, inflection, pauses
- body movement, such as posture, gestures, fidgeting
- physiological responses, such as perspiring, breathing rapidly, blushing
- appearance, such as dress.

In practice, both clients and mental health nurses send many messages and clues through their non-verbal behaviour. It is therefore important that mental health nurses are aware of their own non-verbal body language before they can explore clients' non-verbal behaviour. In practice, however, we may not always be aware of the non-verbal messages that we communicate and, more importantly, how they might affect our interactions and relationship with clients, their families and work colleagues. For example, how often have you said *'It's not what s/he said, but it's the way it was said'* or alternatively someone has said to you *'it's not what you said, but it's how you said it'*?

Effective helpers therefore need to learn 'body language' and how to use it effectively in their interactions with clients, while at the same time being careful not to over-interpret non-verbal communication (Egan, 2010, p.147). Also, when working with clients from different cultural backgrounds, it is important that the mental health nurse is mindful of and sensitive to different practices concerning the use of eye contact and gender, and modify his/her body language accordingly. For example in a number of cultures, including African and Asian, maintaining eye contact with someone who is in a position of authority is likely to be 'interpreted as a demonstration of an equality that is disrespectful and inappropriate' (Sully and Dallas, 2005, p.5).

Non-verbal communication either on its own or together can influence verbal communication in the following ways:

- confirm what is being said verbally, for example when talking about the recent death of her father, the client looked sad and became tearful
- confuse what is being said, for example when telling the client she wanted to hear his story, the nurse kept looking at her watch and fidgeting with her pen

- emphasize what is being said verbally, for example when talking about his anger towards his family for 'forcing him to come into hospital', the client clenched his fist and banged the table
- add intensity to the verbal message, for example when asking for extra medication to stop the voices, the client stood up and put his hands over his ears and shouted 'I want them to stop, I want them to stop.'

The SOLER position

Egan (2010, p.135) identifies certain non-verbal skills summarized in the acronym SOLER that can help the mental health nurse to create the therapeutic space and tune in to what the client is saying. These are:

S: sitting facing the client squarely, at an angle
O: adopting an open posture, arms and legs uncrossed
L: leaning (at times) towards the person
E: maintaining good eye contact, without staring
R: relaxed posture.

As with all interpersonal skills there are a host of things that can hinder the ability to listen attentively. Some of these include:

- distractions in the room, for example noise from TV or radio
- seating, for example uncomfortable place to sit and listen
- temperature of room, for example feeling too cold or too hot and stuffy
- lack of time
- listening to self rather than to client, for example worrying about what you are going to say next, how the client might respond to what you say
- hearing the client talk about things that you find difficult to believe, for example that the voices are instructing them to say or do specific things
- hearing the client talk about very painful experiences that you find very emotionally difficult to hear, for example accounts of physical, psychological or sexual abuse.

We will now look at how using a simple framework can help the listener to structure and organize their conversations with service users, their carers and others who care for and support them.

Listening to verbal communication

Having a framework when listening to a person's story helps to develop 'clinical mindfulness' and assists the listener to organize what the person has said (Bricker et al. 2007, p.25). The following provides a framework to help you focus both your listening and attending with a view to gaining a greater understanding of the person and their story.

Framework for listening and attending to clients

Scenario: Louise

Louise: 'So many things have happened since I was discharged from the day hospital two months ago. I broke up with Harry, my boyfriend, and I moved to a new flat. I really like where I live now, it is smaller but the neighbours are very friendly and helpful. There have been a couple of times when I have been upset and cried a lot, but I know I did the right thing. Harry and I were always arguing about money and his drinking. I used to be afraid that he would hit me. He never did but I do not want to be always afraid. He keeps phoning me, he wants us to get back together. I miss him, [eyes fill up with tears] but I told him I do not want him back. I am much happier now; no more arguments and I am looking forward to lots of things. I am going on holidays with my sister Sharon and her family. They are so good to me.'

Nurse: 'Mm ... mm', leaning forward

- **Experiences:** The client may talk about their experiences, such as what has happened, for example Louise was discharged from the day hospital two months ago. She broke up with Harry, her boyfriend, and moved to a new flat; or what is currently happening in their life, for example Louise is going on holidays with her sister Sharon and her family.
- **Behaviours and patterns of behaviour:** The client may talk about how they behaved or responded to a certain situation(s). The mental health nurse may also be interested in observing how the person is responding while telling his/her story. For example, Harry keeps phoning Louise, he wants them to get back together. She misses him [eyes fill up with tears] but she told him she doesn't want him back.
- **Thoughts and patterns of thinking:** This may include what beliefs they have about themselves, other people, events in their lives, as well as what sense they make of their own and others' behaviours. For example, there have been a couple of times when Louise has been upset and cried a lot, but she believes she has done the right thing. She and Harry were always arguing about money and his drinking. Louise was afraid that he would hit her. He never did, but she doesn't want to be always afraid.
- **Feelings, emotions and moods:** This refers to the client's description of his/her feelings as well as the feelings they are expressing as they tell their story. For example, there have been a couple of times when Louise has been upset and cried a lot; she misses him [eyes fill up with tears] but she told him she does not want him back. She is much happier now.
- **Strengths and resources:** It is important when listening not to focus only on problems; clients also have strengths and resources.

In the above scenario, Louise's strengths include optimism and determination. Other strengths may include humour and friendliness. Resources include, for example, Louise's helpful neighbours and her sister. Other resources may include family, friends and pets.

- **Non-verbal messages:** As previously discussed, there are non-verbal cues, such as facial expressions, body movements and voice tone, which may confirm or deny what is being spoken. Non-verbal behaviours can mean a number of things and caution needs to be used when reading non-verbal behaviour. For example, on observing the client's behaviour of pacing up and down the ward, the mental health nurse might conclude, incorrectly, that the client is anxious or angry, whereas the client later explains that she feels very cold and is walking up and down to keep herself warm.

Source: Adapted from Cully (1992)

The following box consists of a list of behaviours and characteristics that a good listener might demonstrate (Bonham, 2004, p. 21).

The helpful person

- is quiet for most of the conversation, for example allowed you to do most of the talking
- is encouraging, for example demonstrates by their body language that they understand what you are saying. They nod and maintain eye contact without staring and appear interested
- sits or stands in a similar way to you and at a comfortable distance from you, not too close or not too far away.
- appears relaxed to what you are saying, asks to repeat or clarify something to make sure that they understand you
- might sometimes repeat back to you what you have said or summarise what you have said to ensure sure that they understand you
- might convey a sense that they are 'in tune' with what you are saying or experiencing
- does not judge you
- gives you ample time to talk
- leaves you feeling respected

Practice exercise

- Think of a time when you experienced or observed someone to be very helpful in practice.
- Identify which of the above behaviours were used.

Touch

Touch, as a form of non-verbal communication, is an important component of therapeutic communication. In mental health nursing, touch can be used as a means of reassuring and/or breaking down barriers between nurse and client (Gleeson and Higgins, 2009). Touch can be instrumental or procedural, whereby the use of touch is necessary or deliberate, for example administering an injection, taking a client's pulse or blood pressure, bathing or dressing a client. In contrast, 'expressive' touch is non-procedural, more spontaneous and a demonstration of affection, for example holding a client's hand, placing a hand on a client's shoulder (Watson, 1975). As with all communication skills, touch needs to be used with care and respect. Before using touch, mental health nurses need to consider the following points.

- Offer touch respectfully based on the needs of the person as opposed to your own needs. For example the nurse asks the distressed client 'Would you like me to hold your hand?', rather than the nurse initiating holding the client's hand to allay his/her own feelings of discomfort and/or assuming that the client wants or needs to be touched.
- Respect the client's culture, age, ethnicity and gender; for example do not assume that it is OK to touch older clients or children without their permission. Also, in some cultures, it is unacceptable to be touched by people who are not intimate unless it is in the administration of specific physical care.
- Be mindful that clients who experience mental health problems or distress may require special consideration when using touch, as their responses may not always be predictable, for example if a client believes that 'all females want to harm him' it is important that the client's personal space is respected, particularly by female nurses.
- Be aware of your own level of (dis)comfort and be genuine when using touch, for example if you are uncomfortable about using touch then it is better for the client and yourself that you do not force or impose the use of touch without seeking permission.
- Similar to other therapeutic interventions, touch should always be used genuinely and for the client's best interest.

Silence

Being able to be silent and still with the client, particularly when s/he is distressed, demonstrates the ability to be present and with the person (Benner, 2001, p.50). However, this can often evoke some discomfort for both the mental health nurse and the person in distress. As a result, silences can often feel longer than they actually are, especially if the person finds them uncomfortable. Learning to *'sit with'* silence requires practice. One way of learning this skill is for the mental health nurse to practise pausing for five seconds before making an intervention (Stickley and Stacey, 2009). This can help the mental health nurse to refrain from *filling the space* by speaking and yet not allow the silence to be too long to cause possible distress for the client. With time and much practice, learning to be comfortable with silence becomes easier and you will begin to notice the positive impact it has on your interventions. As a therapeutic intervention, the use of silence is a way of communicating respect to the client and, as a result, can convey the following messages, as outlined by Stickley and Stacey (2009, p.51):

- the person is important to you
- you have time for the person
- this interaction is more than a normal conversation
- your interventions are considered
- it is OK to be with the person without feeling the need to do something.

While listening is important, it is usually not enough – the client also wants a response. The following refers to the skills of responding verbally to service users. These are called reflecting and probing skills.

Reflecting skills

Reflecting skills are those skills that help the mental health nurse to focus on the client's perspective, and as such encourage person-centred communication. The main principle in using reflective skills involves identifying the person's core message and offering it back to them in your own words. When using reflective skills, the mental health nurse follows what the client is saying – that is, aiming to be person-centred rather than directing the interaction and imposing what s/he believes to be important, which is nurse-centred communication. Effective use of reflective skills can facilitate exploration, build trust, and communicate acceptance and understanding to the client.

Paraphrasing

Paraphrasing involves expressing the person's core message in your own words. When using paraphrasing, essentially the meaning is not changed but the words are different. Paraphrasing is a valuable tool in that it demonstrates to the client that the mental health nurse is listening and has heard what s/he has said, which can feel very supportive and therefore therapeutic. Paraphrasing can also be used to check clarity and understanding rather than using questions, as illustrated in the following examples.

Example 1

Zoe: Mm. [Pause] I don't know really, I mean, I suppose if there is something you would like me to talk about I would be happy to do that, but as I said, it does feel hard to focus and be here.
Nurse: It seems that it is easier to follow instructions now.

Zoe: Mm, yes, yes, I think that is right. I do not feel very able to think very clearly now, and I have been a bit forgetful over the last couple of weeks. I forgot my keys the other day, which is very unusual for me.

Example 2

Dylan: [with an angry tone] I suppose I felt uncomfortable when my brother asked me to lend him the money. It is not because I do not have the money, I can afford it. I don't know why I was angry, but I, don't want to seem miserly.
Nurse: You felt annoyed when he asked you and didn't want him to think you were mean.
Dylan: Yes, that's right I did feel annoyed ... but I also felt guilty ... He is my youngest brother and he has no one else.

Summarizing

This skill involves offering the client a précis or summary of the information that s/he has given. A summary is essentially a longer paraphrase, however it should not be presented as a list of facts. Summarizing can be a very useful intervention, particularly if the person in distress has given you a lot of information. For the client, hearing a summary of what s/he has said can help to clarify and reassure them that the nurse has heard correctly. It also gives the client the opportunity to correct any misunderstandings, elaborate further as well as hear the main points of their story. When using a summary you may begin by saying something like 'So, to sum up, you have mentioned several issues concerning ... '

Probing skills

Probing skills involve questioning. The most useful forms of questions are open ended and begin with 'when', 'what', 'how', 'who' or 'where'. Asking an open-ended question invites a full descriptive response. For example, if you were exploring a person's experience of hearing voices, you might use some of the following open questions.

Examples of open questions

- When did you first hear the voices?
- How many voices do you hear?
- What do the voices say to you?
- When are the voices loudest?
- Who knows that you hear voices?
- How do you feel, when the voices say ... ?
- What were you doing when the voices became louder?
- What helps you to cope with the voices?

The following illustrates examples of other categories of questions, which can be used when working with clients and their families/carers. These include the following:

- cognitive questions; these focus on the person's thoughts or beliefs
- affective questions; these focus on the person's feelings, mood or affect
- behavioural questions; these focus on the person's behaviour or actions
- time-orientated questions focus on issues relating to time, such as past, present and future.

Other useful open questions

Cognitive questions:	What do you think about when you have a panic attack?
	What did you think would happen when you took the overdose?
	What do you think causes the voices to say those things?
Affective questions:	When you were told about your son's diagnosis, how did you feel?
	How do you feel when the voices call you names?
	How do you feel after you have injured (cut) yourself?
Behavioural questions:	What did you do when you had the panic attack?
	What does your son do when he gets angry?
	What can you do to reduce the stress caused by the voices?
Time-orientated questions:	What did you do in the past that helped you to manage the voices?
	What can you do now to reduce the urge to cut yourself?
	What could you do in the next two hours to keep yourself safe?

Unhelpful questions

Unhelpful questions include the following.

Closed questions

These are questions that limit the other person's options and often only give the option of a 'yes' or 'no' response, for example:

- Did you take your medication?
- Have you seen the doctor?
- Do you hear voices?
- Did you go to the hospital?
- Do you like your parents?

Although closed questions are useful when gathering information, they have limited value and do not encourage dialogue, and as a result reduce the opportunity to engage with the client. Overuse of closed questions can also set up a pattern of 'questions and answers', which can be hard to break.

Other questions, which are unhelpful in encouraging dialogue and person-centred communication, include the following.

Leading questions

As the name suggests, these questions involve imposing your own perspective or being suggestive, for example 'I don't think you are very happy with your husband?' rather than, 'How do you feel towards your husband?', which encourages person-centred communication rather than nurse-led communication.

Multiple questions

These involve asking two or more questions at once, for example 'What did the doctor say when you told him about your panic attacks; did he suggest reviewing your medication and did he refer you to the anxiety management group?' It is not surprising that this can be confusing and unhelpful for the client. In addition, when the client answers, the mental health nurse will not know which question the client has answered.

Either/or questions

These questions are both leading and restrictive because the options put forward are what the nurse has chosen and, as with multiple questions, they involve two questions, for example 'What do you want to do, go for a walk or attend the anxiety management group?'

The 'why' question

The 'why' question tends to invite an answer rather than a description or an exploration. In addition, the use of 'why' may appear interrogative and as a result may evoke a defensive answer from the person. For example, how might *you* feel and respond if you were asked the following 'why' questions:

'Why were you late?'; 'Why did you say that?' Such questions may cause the person to feel defensive and/or irritated. Therefore, it may not be surprising that the following why question might evoke such a limited response:

Nurse: 'Why didn't you take your medication?'

Client: 'Because I forgot.'

Poorly timed questions

As with all interpersonal skills, timing is critical to asking effective questions. For example, if a client who is very distressed relates having an argument with his father and the nurses asks, 'What did you say that might have contributed to the argument?' it is unlikely that the client will be willing to explore his own behaviour at this particular time and may feel unheard by the nurse.

Learning to ask questions without using 'why' can be challenging and require patience and plenty of practice. The following illustrates some practice examples of 'why' questions and how these questions might be asked more effectively.

'Why' questions	Alternative phrasings
Why didn't you take your medication?	What stopped you from taking your medication?
Why did you take an overdose?	What made you take an overdose?
Why did you discharge yourself from hospital?	What happened that led you to discharge yourself?
Why do you get anxious?	What do you think causes you to feel anxious?
Why did you say that?	What made you say that?

Using skills in practice

As with most acquired skills, learning how to use the different interpersonal skills and use them effectively takes time, practice, motivation, and the courage to make mistakes and *be imperfect*. There are no verbal formulas or magical sentences that will solve clients' problems. Equally, there are no set 'right or wrong' or 'good or bad' communication skills. Instead, there are useful and non-useful skills and interventions. Learning how to communicate effectively in practice will present mental health nurses with different learning opportunities and challenges; but in order for lifelong learning to take place we strongly encourage you to take some time to think about each interaction, your communication skills and their therapeutic effectiveness. The following questions provide a simple framework to help you evaluate your interactions in clinical practice.

Practice exercise

Take some time to think about a recent interaction that took place during your clinical practice. Reflect on the following questions and jot down your thoughts, ideas and feelings in your journal. Try to be as specific as possible in your answers, as illustrated below. You may also wish to spend some time reflecting on your answers with a colleague or your mentor.

Reflective questions

1   What did I like best about my use of interpersonal skills?
    For example: I liked best that I listened even though at times I was tempted to ask a question.

2   What did I like least about my use of interpersonal skills?
    For example: I liked least that I asked a closed and leading question a few times.

3   If I were to do this interaction again, what would I do differently and why?
    For example: I would summarize what the client said to me. This would have helped me to stop worrying that I was going to forget what the client said, and as a result I didn't listen to the client.

4   What have I learnt from this interaction?
    For example: I learnt that I need to practise the use of summarizing.

Conclusion

This chapter has outlined the different verbal and non-verbal skills that are used in mental health practice. These interpersonal skills can be learnt and used in various clinical encounters. It is not enough, however, simply to learn communication skills and techniques; they must be integrated into your own style of working as a mental health nurse. As with all new learning, this will require time, practise and a willingness to be open to feedback from clients and colleagues about your use of different skills and their therapeutic impact in practice. While we hope that this chapter is useful to you in developing your repertoire of communication skills, it is not intended to be the only source of learning. Nevertheless, we hope it provides a useful framework to identify and clarify what skills you are using and, more importantly, to consider its usefulness in developing your communication skills as a mental health nurse.

Reflective questions

1 What type of questions should *not* be used or at best should be used sparingly, and for what reasons?
2 When using the skill of listening in your practice, identify three things you found rewarding and challenging?
3 What three communication skills do you want to improve and for what reasons?
4 How would you explain to a colleague that 'why' questions should be used sparingly?

2 Values, culture and evidence-based communication

Introduction

Mental health nurses' ability to deliver care using the best possible evidence is a necessary, but insufficient component of their practice. It is increasingly recognized that values are as central to mental health practice as evidence (Woodbridge and Fulford, 2004; Seedhouse, 2005; Cooper, 2009). The values and skills mental health nurses hold shape their practice and, when considered alongside people's cultural differences and evidence, may contribute to providing care that fosters people's recovery and sense of wellbeing.

In 1952, Hildegard Peplau, an American psychiatric nurse wrote a seminal work on interpersonal relations in nursing (Peplau, 1952). In this book, Peplau argued that effective communication skills were central to sound interpersonal skills and fundamental to the role of mental health nurses. This view is supported by more recent work (Hewitt et al., 2009). In this chapter, we will examine values, culture and evidence-based communication styles designed to foster recovery in people living with mental distress and promote their sense of wellbeing through the adoption of positive mental health nursing.

Learning outcomes

By the end of this chapter, you should be better able to:

1 explain what is meant by values, and cultural- and evidence-based communication styles
2 understand how to demonstrate these styles in your practice
3 evaluate, in partnership with people using services, the effectiveness of these styles.

Values-based communication

Taking Fulford's (2004) definition of values-based practice as a template, the mental health nurse who uses a values-based communication style will recognize that different and potentially conflicting values may be evident in working therapeutically with service users. Values-based practice is a core component of the Department of Health's (2004) Essential Shared Capabilities required of the mental health workforce, of mental health nurses at the point of registration, as outlined in the Chief Nursing Officers' *Reviews of Mental Health Nursing* (DH, 2006; Scottish Executive, 2006) and the Nursing and Midwifery Council's (NMC, 2008) learning outcomes for mental health nurses and the new NMC standards for pre-registration nursing. A review of evidence of research with mental health service users demonstrates the importance they attach to encountering mental health nurses who hold the values that will assist service users achieve recovery (Bee et al., 2007).

The National Framework of Values for Mental Health is underpinned by three key principles:

1   recognition of the role of values alongside evidence in mental health practice
2   raising awareness of how values impact practice
3   respect for diversity, i.e. that all mental health practitioners will uphold equality and not discriminate on grounds like gender, sexual orientation, age, degree of ability, religion, race, ethnicity or culture.

Using Fulford's (2004) approach, a mental health nurse who practices values-based communication will be:

- person-centred – puts the service user and carers at the heart of their practice
- recovery focused – practice empowering service users to find their road towards recovery
- work in partnership with others as required
- dynamic – will be able and willing to change communication style where required
- reflective – will examine regularly their communication style
- balanced – will recognize positive and negative values inherent in their communication style
- relationship focused – will recognize the contribution of sound communication skills to fostering therapeutic relationships.

A helpful starting point for a consideration of the values that may underpin your practice as a mental health nurse when communicating with service users involves reflecting upon several ideas and questions (Cooper, 2009, p.3):

- what are values?
- how to identify your personal values
- how to identify and respect the values of others
- why are values important in helping professions?
- how to develop and apply values to mental health nursing practice
- how to identify and resolve a conflict of values.

Woodbridge and Fulford (2004) wrote a seminal report on values-based practice. In this report, the authors describe the skills required of a

Table 2.1 Applying the skills required of a values-based practitioner to mental health nursing communication (after Woodbridge and Fulford, 2004, p.20)

Skills required of values-based practitioner	Description	Application by mental health nurse practising values-based communication
Awareness	Recognizing the values that might be present in a particular situation	If you are communicating with a service user, check how they like to be addressed, for example as a patient, service user, a person with lived experience of mental illness
Reasoning	Using logical and sound processes to explore the values behind practice	Analyse the components of the communication style you use and identify the values being demonstrated at each stage. For example, if you can record an interaction with a service user, consider the language you use and ask your clinical supervisor to listen and provide feedback
Knowledge	Understanding the values and facts relevant to a situation	Reflect on the values and evidence behind the choice of communication, for example consider how your choice of language might communicate your values. Does your use of the term mental illness suggest that you are adopting a biomedical approach?
Communication	The interpersonal skills, combined with awareness, reasoning and knowledge to resolve conflicts	Identify the values and evidence-based communication styles that resolve conflict (see Chapter 9 and in particular use the conflict-provoking self-assessment tool to reflect on your communication style)

values-based practitioner. Table 2.1 shows how these skills could be applied to a values-based communication style for mental health nursing.

Culture-based communication

An important part of values-based communication is demonstrating cultural sensitivity, competence and capability. Mental health nurses have an important role in delivering equality in mental health services through culturally capable practice. However, there is widespread evidence that people from black and ethnic minority groups do not feel that the care they receive is equal, equitable and sensitive to their needs (DH, 2005).

Culture is a shared set of learned behaviours, values, beliefs, norms, assumptions, perceptions, customs, social interactions and the world-view of a particular group (Allot, 2005). A mental health nurse who communicates in a culturally capable style is likely to:

- increase his/her own multicultural understanding – be aware of his/her own biases
- assess the extent to which people are orientated to their culture, for example not all people belonging to the same ethnic group will be orientated to the same culture
- explore/assess how culture relates to thoughts, feelings and behaviour
- demonstrate cultural sensitivity through understanding different experiences
- respect cultural norms in communication styles
  - be aware of and avoid stereotyping
  - ask, listen and respect
  - be flexible – accommodate individual needs as far as possible
  - respect and accept diversity.

(Callaghan, 2006)

Mental health nurses often work in multicultural settings and interact with people from different cultural and ethnic groups. People within these groups often behave and communicate in different ways. When working with people from different cultural and ethnic groups the following communication issues may arise.

- Rules – groups have different rules for communication, e.g. maintaining eye contact may be offensive to some cultural groups.
- Language – different groups often have their own language and dialect, e.g. the use of different terms for mental illness.
- Motivation – factors that drive communication such as rules and rituals may vary, e.g. people may defer to you as they perceive that having a professional status gives you a more prominent place than them in a hierarchy.
- Ideals and values – different beliefs underpin communication, e.g. people may not talk about mental illness in terms of symptoms they are experiencing, but in terms of their beliefs in the causes of the illness.
- Cooperation and competition – communication may be driven by these goals, e.g. if people wish to cooperate with you they may be less challenging to your ideas and beliefs than if they wish to compete with you.
- Collectivism and individualism – communication may be directed at promoting the collective or the individual good, e.g. people from so-called collectivist societies like China or India may attribute their successes to external events and their failures to their individual weaknesses.

- Greetings and other rituals – different groups have different rituals and ways of greeting each other, e.g. handshakes, kissing.

(Callaghan, 2006)

Different cultural and ethnic groups have different styles of communication. The following issues may arise when communicating with people from such groups.

- Cultural context of language – the influence of culture on language varies, e.g. people may be more or less deferential depending on their view of your place in their hierarchy.
- Self-disclosure – the meaning, use and nature of self-disclosure varies among different groups, e.g. disclosing personal information to a stranger.
- The preservation of face (that is, not humiliating someone in front of others) is important in certain groups, e.g. Chinese and Japanese people.
- The use and meaning of silence varies with different cultures, e.g. silence may be a sign of passive aggression.
- Varieties of truthfulness (that is, respect for truth varies in different cultures), e.g. in order to save face, people may be less than truthful to you.
- Complimenting and responding – may take different forms, e.g. compliments may be expressed in a general sense, rather than individually.
- Non-verbal behaviour has different meanings in different cultures, e.g. using handshakes or physical contact when interacting with others.

(Callaghan, 2006)

So far in this chapter we have outlined the importance of values-based practice and cultural sensitivity to your work as mental health nurse when communicating with service users and others. We believe that reflecting upon the values and cultural norms that lie behind your practice and the behaviour of the service users for whom you care is fundamental to communicating effectively.

Practice exercise

Consider the different ways in which people from different cultural groups communicate with you. Now identify examples from your own practice where you were communicating with people from a culture different from your own. Answer the following questions.

- What were the challenges you faced?
- How did you respond to these challenges?
- What was the outcome of your encounter?

In the next section of this chapter, we will examine how basing your communication style on the best possible evidence will augment the values and cultural-based approaches to practice to produce an optimal level of practice.

Evidence-based communication

During the Qing dynasty in 18th-century China, several scholars developed an interest in gaining knowledge from a type of methodology that they called *kaozheng*, or 'practising evidential research'. This principle was based on painstaking evaluation of data based on high standards of rigour and precision. The aim of *kaozheng* scholars was to base their views on facts established from empirical evidence (Spence, 1991, p.103). This is an early example of the philosophy driving much of evidence-based practice (EBP) in mental health nursing today. In a contemporary view, EBP is defined as 'the conscientious, explicit and judicious use of current best evidence in making decisions about the care of individual patients' (Sackett et al., 1996, p.71).

The notion that mental health nursing communication should be based on the best possible evidence is sound, but it is unclear at what point is enough evidence gathered to justify one approach over another. The integration of clinical acumen with current best evidence will improve mental health nurses' communication. However, health problems are not neatly resolved by recourse to evidence. Questions relating to the care of patients are not all answered by science; health care is at the interface of many disciplines, and to understand fully the experience of health and ill health, we need to draw from many types of evidence, such as:

- evidence derived from empirical research
- systematic and other reviews of such research
- clinical guidelines such as those published by the National Institute for Health and Clinical Excellence (NICE)
- expert opinion
- the views, preferences and values of people using, and those providing, mental health services.

There is value in using the best possible evidence as this may lead to:

- improved care
- directing resources cost-effectively
- increased professionalism
- better partnerships with people using services.

With the above caveats in mind, in this section we shall consider the evidence base for various communication styles that are of use to mental health nurses. In particular, we explore and illustrate what works, for whom and under what therapeutic conditions.

Skills for evidence-based practice

Gray (1997) argues that patient care decisions are based on evidence, values and resources. He goes on to state that the optimum use of resources will be evidence-based. According to Gray (1997, p.2) the evidence-based practitioner requires several skills:

- an ability to define criteria such as effectiveness, safety and acceptability
- an ability to find articles on the effectiveness, safety and acceptability of a new test or treatment
- an ability to assess the quality of evidence
- an ability to assess whether the result of research can be generalized to the whole population from which the sample was drawn
- an ability to assess whether the results of the research are applicable to a 'local' population.

Table 2.2 outlines how mental health nurses can demonstrate these skills when considering the evidence for different communication styles in routine clinical practice using Gray's approach.

Practice exercise

You are working in a community mental health team and are due to meet with Jane, a service user whom you have been caring for in the past three weeks. Jane often challenges you on your communication style and tells you that it does not suit her. However, you have read a recently published research paper that supports the style you have been using with Jane. Reflect on the application of evidence-based communication skills shown in the third column of Table 2.2. Now consider how you might communicate differently with Jane while upholding the research you have read.

Having considered the skills required to make sense of evidence that you retrieve to help you in your pursuit of evidence-based communication, we now examine the evidence for different forms of therapeutic communication.

Therapeutic communication: what works, for whom and under what conditions?

Effective communication and interpersonal skills are considered central to mental health nurses' ability to form a sound therapeutic alliance with

Table 2.2 Applying the skills required of an evidence-based practitioner to mental health nursing communication

Skills required of an evidence-based practitioner	Description	Application by mental health nurse practising evidence-based communication
Ability to define criteria such as effectiveness, safety and acceptability	Understanding the meaning of effectiveness, safety and acceptability	Identify the evidence behind chosen communication style, consider the safety of this style and its acceptability to service users For example, check whether using eye contact is acceptable to the service user
Ability to find articles on the effectiveness, safety and acceptability of a new test or treatment	Knowing how to find articles on the effectiveness, safety and acceptability of a new test or treatment	Select the chosen communication style and review published evidence as to its effectiveness, safety and acceptability For example, if you use the person's first name without their permission, will they find it offensive?
Ability to assess the quality of evidence	Evaluating the quality of published evidence	Check with the service user whether the evidence you have read matches their preferred style of communication
Ability to assess whether the result of research can be generalized to the whole population from which the sample was drawn	Understanding how the results of published research from a small population can be applied to a larger one	When you find that a particular style of communication works with one person, consider using it again with others
Ability to assess whether the results of the research are applicable to a 'local' population	Understanding how the results of published research from a global population can be applied to a local one	Discuss the latest research with the service user and check their view as to how it might apply to them

people for whom they care. An effective therapeutic relationship is shown to improve the care you can offer to service users. Table 2.3 shows core skills and values that you might find helpful in communicating with service users.

Table 2.3 Core attitudes, values and skills in developing, maintaining and ending therapeutic encounters (Myles and Richards, 2006)

Core attitudes and values
Communicate respect
Communicate empathy
Communicate genuineness

Setting clinical boundaries
Behaviours – do not give presents, make sexual contact or communicate in a sexual manner, or reveal highly personal information about yourself
Language – profanities, i.e. swear words, should be avoided by both user and nurse
Touch – avoid any touching beyond a handshake
Space – the healthcare setting is usually the most appropriate place to meet. If you work with the person in another setting be mindful of safety issues and the need to respect the fact that you are a guest in the person's setting

Developing the therapeutic encounter
Check the person's name and how they like to be addressed
Introduce yourself
State your role
State the aim of the interaction
State the time allotted
Agree ground rules for acceptable and unacceptable behaviours (see below)

Maintaining the therapeutic encounter
Use non-verbal skills – e.g. suitable posture, eye contact, facial expression, tone of voice
Listen actively – do not interrupt, pay attention, be non-judgemental, do not give direct advice, clarify anything that is not clear, provide enough time, do not undermine the person's problem
Use verbal skills – paraphrase, i.e. repeat back to the person what they have said, reflect on the feelings that may underpin any verbal statement, be empathic, i.e. convey your understanding of the impact of what the person is saying
Protect confidential information – however, be mindful that you will need to breach confidentiality if it is in the person's or the public's interest to do so on the grounds that there may be harm to the person or others. The NMC Code of Professional Conduct (see Chapter 7) provides guidance on this issue. For child protection issues check the Department of Health Guidelines on www.dh.gov.uk

Ending the therapeutic encounter
Prepare the person for the end of the alliance
End the alliance in a manner that does not leave unresolved tensions or problems
End when the goals agreed at the beginning have been achieved
Leave the person feeling optimistic and hopeful

Practice exercise

Read the following extract from a therapeutic encounter between David, a mental health nurse, and Joseph, a service user.

David: greeting Joe with a hug: 'Bloody cold today Joe isn't it?'
Joseph: 'My name is not Joe I'm not here to talk about the weather.'
David: 'Oh, forgive me. How do you like to be addressed?'
Joseph: 'I prefer Joseph.'
David: 'Joseph it is. I'm David, a mental health nurse in the team. I asked to see you today to discuss your progress with the homework task I set three weeks ago. It should take no longer than an hour. Is this OK with you?'
Joseph: 'I was working on the task, but I fell in the snow and almost broke my leg.'
David: showing concern: 'I imagine that was painful; I remember when it happened once to me and I could not concentrate on anything for ages afterwards.'
Joseph: 'Yes it was very painful. And I could not . . .'
David: 'Finish the homework, yes I guess that was difficult.'
Joseph: 'No, I finished the task, it just took longer than I expected.'
David: 'It took longer than expected?'
Joseph: 'Yes, I'm not cut out for this sort of thing. I feel I'm back in school.'
David: 'Was school difficult for you?'
Joseph: 'Yes, somewhat, I did not get good grades. The teachers called me stupid.'
David: 'I guess there are stupider things.'
Joseph: 'That's not how I felt then, or now, as a matter of fact.'
David: 'No problem, I'd like to move on to discussing your medication.'
Joseph: 'Oh OK. What about it?'
David: 'Just checking it's OK.'
Joseph: 'Yes it's fine.'
David: 'Well if that's all, we'll leave it there until next time.'

Now consider the core skills and values in developing, maintaining and ending the therapeutic encounter shown in Table 2.3.

Identify in the encounter between David and Joseph examples of good and poor communication techniques that David uses.

The content shown in Table 2.3 has remained relatively unchallenged as exemplars of effective styles of communication. However, in *Talking with Acutely Psychotic People*, Bowers and colleagues (2009) describe ways that expert mental health nurses working in acute inpatient psychiatric wards communicate with people for whom they care (see Figure 2.1).

Practice exercise

Below are examples of communicative actions taken by mental health nurses that Bowers and colleagues (2009) report.

(continued)

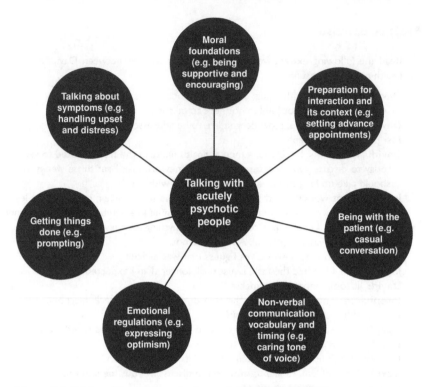

Figure 2.1 Talking with acutely psychotic people (Bowers et al., 2009)

- expressing empathy
- communicating respect
- a caring tone of voice.

Now give examples from what you have learnt so far in this chapter of how you would apply these skills in practice.

Therapeutic encounters between mental health nurses and service users occur during formal psychotherapeutic interventions, or through 'routine' encounters. In their comprehensive review of what works for whom in psychotherapy, Roth and Fonagy (2005) report that developing, sustaining and ending the therapeutic encounter successfully appeared consistent irrespective of client group or mental health condition.

In the final part of this chapter we consider the communication styles that foster recovery in people experiencing mental distress.

Fostering recovery and wellbeing through therapeutic communication

We have established firmly that sound therapeutic relationships help foster people's recovery from mental distress. Recovery involves helping people with mental health problems live 'meaningful and satisfying lives' (Shepherd et al., 2009). Recovery approaches are currently being adopted in many mental health services in different parts of the world and are central to the DH's recently published mental health strategy *No Health without Mental Health* (DH, 2011). In addition to fostering recovery, it is helpful to consider how promoting wellbeing aids people's recovery (see Carson and Gordon, 2010). Mental health nurses can contribute to people's recovery by adopting a recovery-orientated approach to their practice. They can have a key role in promoting wellbeing, but both approaches require a shift in nurses' attitudes, values and beliefs, as well as attending to aspects of their own mental health and wellbeing. In the remaining part of this chapter, we outline the key communications skills mental health nurses might find helpful in adopting the 'Ten top tips for recovery-orientated practice' as shown in Table 2.4.

Studies on the effects of wellbeing on general health are gathering momentum. The positive psychology approach that Seligman and others advocate (Seligman et al., 2006) coalesces nicely with the happiness approach that economists like Layard (2005) report are crucial to sound mental health. In Lyubomirsky's view, there are 12 ways to improve wellbeing:

1 cultivating optimism
2 avoiding over-thinking and social comparison
3 practising acts of kindness
4 nurturing relationships
5 developing coping strategies
6 learning to forgive
7 doing more of what engages you
8 savouring life's joys
9 committing to goals
10 practising religion or spirituality
11 taking care of your body
12 expressing gratitude.

(Lyubomirsky, 2008)

While at first glance these may seem a little bit righteous, these ideas are being tested in research. A new approach to mental health nursing – the positive approach based on Aristotle's concept of *eudaimonia*, or human flourishing, and based on Lyubomirsky's 12 ways – could be incorporated by you in helping people rediscover their sense of personal wellbeing. The following is a set of reflective questions that may help you in this pursuit.

Table 2.4 Communication skills central to recovery-orientated practice (Shepherd et al., 2009)

Ten top tips for recovery-orientated practice	Communication skills required of mental health nurses
Listen actively to help the person make sense of their mental health problems	Active listening. Do not interrupt, pay attention, be non-judgemental, do not give direct advice, clarify anything that is not clear, provide enough time, do not undermine the person's situation
Help the person identify and prioritize *their* personal goals for recovery	Brainstorm all possible goals and help person rank-order chosen goals
Demonstrate a belief in the person's existing strengths and resources in relation to the pursuit of personal goals	Acknowledge and reinforce strengths and resources
Identify examples from your own 'lived experience', or that of other service users, which inspires and validates their hopes	Use empathic statements, for example 'When I faced a similar issue, doing exercise helped me get through it'
Pay particular attention to the importance of goals that take the person out of the sick role and enable them to contribute actively to the lives of others	
Identify non-mental health resources – friends, contacts, organizations – relevant to the achievement of their goals	Provide tips on how to navigate and access these resources, for example give people a list of local amenities that they can access
Encourage self-management of mental health problems (by providing information or reinforcing coping strategies)	Consider informative interventions (see Chapter five). For example, you might provide a handout showing different ways of coping with stress
Discuss what sort of therapeutic interventions the person wants, respect their wishes where possible	Outline possible interventions to help them on their way if necessary, for example if the person likes exercise then you could recommend a brisk walk each day for 30 minutes
Behave at all times so as to convey an attitude of respect for the person and a desire for an equal partnership in working together, indicating a willingness to go the extra mile	See the sections on values and culture-based communication above for helpful hints
While accepting the future is uncertain and setbacks happen, continue to express support for the possibility of achieving these self-defined goals thereby maintaining hope and positive expectations	Continue to acknowledge and reinforce the hopeful journey the person is taking towards their recovery

> **Reflections on communicating positive mental health nursing**
>
> Ask yourself:
>
> - what examples can I recall from practice that have helped people lead meaningful and satisfying lives that promote their sense of wellbeing?
> - what actions have I taken with people to show that I am communicating in a values, culture and evidence-based manner?
> - when talking with people challenged by psychotic episodes, what actions have helped me to foster therapeutic communication?
> - when I consider a recent therapeutic encounter, how did I develop, maintain and end this encounter in a way that transformed the experience for me and the person with whom I was working?
> - what can I learn from actions to promote my own sense of wellbeing that might help people in my care?

Conclusion

In this chapter, we argue that therapeutic communication requires mental health nurses to demonstrate a values-, culture- and evidence-based approach to practice, an approach that we call 'positive mental health nursing'. It requires mental health nurses to apply the art, craft and science of nursing and other disciplines to consider what works for whom, where and under what conditions the practice of mental health nursing might flourish. It is likely, even in a world where new roles in mental health emerge to challenge them, that mental health nurses will be called upon to show that mental health nursing still matters. The chance to adopt positive mental health nursing gives nurses an opportunity to show that they can help people lead meaningful and satisfying lives and promote their sense of wellbeing.

Reflective questions

1 Consider Fulford's (2004) seven features of values-based communication. How can you demonstrate these in your everyday work?
2 What five skills might indicate to others that you are an evidence-based practitioner?
3 Why are the core attitudes, values and skills in developing, maintaining and ending therapeutic encounters central to how you communicate with others in a therapeutic setting?
4 What skills might you use to foster the recovery of people in your care?

3 Reflection and communication

Introduction

Reflection is an important component in the process of becoming a mental health nurse as well as a recommended element of continuing professional development post-registration. Its value in contributing to mental health nurses' learning and development is recognized and supported by the nursing profession. This chapter will examine the concept of reflection, its usefulness in enhancing nurses' learning, as well as its value in developing the skills required for effective communication. We will also outline various strategies that aim to help the mental health nurse to develop his/her ability to become a more reflective communicator in clinical practice.

Learning outcomes

By the end of this chapter, you should be better able to:

1 Describe the concept of reflection
2 Demonstrate an understanding of how reflection can be used to enhance learning
3 Demonstrate how reflection can be used to enhance effective communication in clinical practice
4 Use reflection in clinical practice

Understanding reflection – what is it?

The concepts of reflection, reflective practice and the development of reflective practitioners have received much attention and debate within the nursing literature. However, issues relating to reflection are complex. These issues are further compounded by the fact that there are numerous definitions throughout the literature, which are often used in different contexts as though there was a shared agreed meaning of the terminology used. It is therefore important to be explicit about what is understood by the term reflection and, more importantly, how it is used in practice. Reflection is a difficult concept to define. At its simplest, reflection generally refers to a form of thinking. It is essentially a process of thinking about an experience to promote understanding and learning. Reflection or, to be more precise, 'to reflect' is a purposeful activity which involves the person 'recapturing their experience, thinking about it, mulling it over and evaluating it' (Boud et al., 1985, p.19). This deliberative activity also entails the person's ability to examine his/her thoughts, feelings and actions, and think deeply about their experience in order to gain new ideas and perspectives (Atkins and Murphy, 1993). Reflection therefore requires the person to look backwards and to project forwards to the future, which involves the skills of recall and reasoning (Jarvis, 1992). In this way, reflection aims 'to build bridges between past and present experiences to determine future nursing action' (Durgahee, 1998, p.158). The following example illustrates how making links between the past, present and future enhanced a specific piece of learning for the mental health nurse.

Clinical scenario

John, a second-year student, listened attentively to Paul as he talked about his experience of hearing voices. John used the probing skills of open questioning and paraphrasing to try to gain a better understanding of Paul's story and distress. Paul described what the voices said to him and how the voices had interfered with every aspect of his life since he left university more than 20 years ago. When the interaction ended, Paul thanked John and said 'it was really good to talk; I don't think I have ever said so much, the staff don't usually ask me talk about my voices'.

Later that day John discussed his interventions and their effectiveness with his mentor. While thinking more about his interaction with Paul, John recalled his first interaction with Paul over six months ago during his first clinical placement. He remembered feeling very anxious and unskilled. In fact, he sometimes made excuses to end the conversation, as he was afraid that he might say the wrong thing and upset Paul. Being aware of his behaviours in the past prompted John to feel embarrassed and uncomfortable, yet he decided to disclose this to his mentor. His mentor acknowledged John's recent awareness and subsequent learning. John now recognized that he had acquired knowledge and different communication skills since then, and as a result, he felt more confident and effective as a mental health nurse. His mentor commented that his interventions were appropriate and, more importantly, that the client had experienced them as effective. John was pleased with his learning to date. However, he also recognized that he had much more to learn; in particular, he wanted to acquire additional skills and strategies that would help Paul to manage his voices more effectively.

Learning by thinking about an experience is not a new concept (Burns and Bulman, 2000). In the 1930s, John Dewey, an American educationalist, provided one of the first explanations of reflection. He viewed reflection as the stepping back from a challenging experience, which allowed the person to think about the experience and then create a more comprehensive plan of action (Dewey, 1933). However, it was not until several decades later that reflection took on a greater role and importance in professional practice. During this time, a number of writers developed their ideas of reflection and presented various definitions of reflection relevant to nursing. The most frequently described in the literature are those of Schön (1983, 1987); Boyd and Fales (1983); Boud et al. (1985); Gibbs (1988) and Johns (2000).

Since the 1980s, the concept of reflection has gained increasing momentum in nursing practice and nurse education throughout the UK. In clinical practice learning through reflection 'has become more prevalent because of the processes of change in contemporary society' (Jarvis et al., 2003, p.9). Also within many pre-registration nurse education programmes, learning outcomes relating to reflection are an explicit learning requirement and form the basis for many formative assessments (Hannigan, 2001). Similar to other practice-based professions, reflection has become a valued and integral component in the learning, acquisition and assessment of knowledge and skills in nursing. In nursing, the use of reflection was influenced by Donald Schön's (1983, 1987) seminal work *The Reflective Practitioner*. He identified two separate types of reflection, described as reflection-on-action and reflection-in-action, the latter usually being carried out more by experienced practitioners. Reflection-in-action refers to the reflective thinking that occurs in the process of an experience (Schön, 1987). For example, during a conversation with a client about different anxiety management strategies that he could use when discharged, the nurse observed that the client was clenching his fist as he answered with monosyllabic responses. At the time, the nurse considered possible explanations for the client's non-verbal behaviour; however she decided not to comment on it until later. Refection-on-action is the retrospective contemplation of practice taken by the nurse to clarify knowledge used in practice. As such, reflection-in action refers to what is happening in the present, whereas reflection-on action is about what happened in the past.

The value of reflection

Many nurse educators and clinicians advocate the use of reflection as a potent and valuable teaching and learning method, which aims to enhance the following:

- integrate theory with practice, thereby narrowing the theory – practice gap (Nicholl and Higgins, 2004)
- promote critical thinking and problem solving (Cotton, 2001)
- maximize clinical learning (Wong et al., 1997)
- facilitate new understanding and learning of nursing (Boud et al., 1985)
- develop professional practice (Somerville and Keeling, 2004)
- improve patient care (Cooke and Matarasso, 2005).

Notwithstanding the above, there is a lack of empirical evidence to support these claims, particularly with regard to how the use of reflection improves patient care (Burns and Bulman, 2000). Much of the extensive literature on reflection and reflective practice is theoretical, descriptive and anecdotal. However, in recent years there has been an increase in research studies, albeit that few relate specifically to reflection and mental health nursing (Platzer et al.,

2000; Glaze 2001; Mantzoukas and Jasper 2004; Nicholl and Higgins 2004; McGrath and Higgins 2006). The mental health nurse needs to be mindful of such limitations when considering reflection in the context of clinical practice and the development of reflective practice. Nonetheless, we believe that the use of reflection in practice can offer the potential for professional and personal development, and learning. However, we are also aware that for learning to occur, the mental health nurse will require structure, guidance and support as well as an openness to use different strategies that foster the ongoing development of reflective skills and reflective practice.

The reflective process

Regardless of what particular model is used, there are three essential stages to the process of reflection (Atkins and Murphy, 1993). These stages consist of the following: first, there is a trigger event or experience and an awareness of uncomfortable feelings or thoughts; secondly a critical analysis of the event, feelings, thoughts or responses; finally, development of a new perspective.

The following specific skills are also required for reflection to take place: self-awareness of one's thinking, feeling and behaviour; critical analysis; synthesis; and evaluation.

Learning how to use the latter higher-order thinking processes will take time and the use of different reflective strategies, which aim to enhance the process of reflective learning and practice. These reflective strategies will now be described.

Models of reflection

There are several reflective models described in the nursing literature, for example Gibbs's (1988) reflective cycle and Rolfe et al.'s (2001) framework for reflective practice. Models of reflection provide different frameworks, which inform and guide how reflection is understood and used in practice. Using a reflective model provides a strategy for intentional reflection on issues that are relevant to clinical practice.

A model of reflection may also:

- provide a useful tool to encourage a deeper, more meaningful exploration of nursing practice
- help the nurse to integrate their knowledge, personal and professional experience
- be adapted to meet the mental health nurse's specific learning needs
- be used by both the novice and expert nurse
- be used alone or with others, for example you may chose to use one of the following reflective models as a framework while writing your reflective diary; alternatively, you could choose a model to stimulate your thinking when sharing your reflections with others in a reflective practice group.

For the purpose of this chapter, we have chosen Gibbs's (1988) reflective model to illustrate how it can be used to reflect on a specific experience or event.

Gibbs's model of reflection

Gibbs's (1988) reflective model provides a simple framework for reflection. It comprises three main stages of reflection, which are cyclical and include the following description and analysis of the experience, as well as the learning acquired from reflecting on the experience. This model also identifies specific questions to facilitate the nurse's ability to think more deeply about a specific experience or event. This in turn helps the nurse to make sense of his/her experience. The model also includes a conclusion that considers other alternatives, along with an action plan to guide the practitioner in the event of a similar situation arising again. It can be used on its own or as a structured framework when writing your reflective journal. The following example illustrates Louise's, a first-year student, use of Gibbs's model to reflect on a specific experience that occurred during her second clinical placement.

Using Gibbs's model of reflection

Description: What happened?
Feelings: What were you thinking and feeling?
Evaluation: What was good and bad about the experience?

It was my first day on the ward. I was excited although a little nervous. This ward was the older adult ward. I was afraid that the client would not take what I said seriously because I look so young. The staff nurse asked me to talk to Mrs Gray, a 70-year-old lady. She had just seen her doctor. I introduced myself and commented on the photos of her lovely grandchildren. She reminded me of my Nan. I felt less nervous and was talking away. I asked her about her grandchildren, their names and ages. Mrs Gray told me their names, ages and what they were doing. Her face lit up as she talked about them. She suddenly became tearful and started crying uncontrollably. She kept saying 'I am going to forget them, I won't know them any more.' I did not know what to say; I wanted to give her a hug but I did not think it was the right thing to do. I just stood and held her hand. The staff nurse came into the room and gently asked Mrs Gray what was wrong. She said the doctor had just told her 'she was losing her memory'. Using listening skills and encouraging prompts, for example 'tell me more', the staff nurse encouraged Mrs Gray to talk. She talked for a long time about what she had been told, her fears and what this meant for her. I tried to listen, but I felt embarrassed for upsetting her.

I felt so stupid in front of the staff nurse.

Thoughts: I did something wrong.

The staff nurse would think I was uncaring and stupid.

Feelings: I felt upset for making Mrs Gray cry.

I think it was good that I tried to listen to Mrs Gray.

I resisted my need to hug her.

I wasn't aware of the client's needs and just started talking without thinking and using my observation skills.

I wasn't listening actively all of the time; I was distracted, worrying about what the staff nurse might think of me.

Analysis: What sense can you make of the experience?

Mrs Gray was upset after receiving this distressing news. I didn't know this and my comments about her grandchildren triggered her feelings. She was upset and frightened. I felt upset because the client was upset; I wanted to make it better for her. I liked this client, she reminded me of Nan. I know that I talk a lot and very quickly when I am nervous. The doctor should have told the nursing staff what he said to Mrs Gray, so we or I could have been more prepared for her response.

Conclusion: What else could you have done?

Be more 'tuned in' to the client's body language and other signs that might indicate the client's feelings.

Action plan: If it arose again, what would you do?

Ask her about her conversation with her doctor, for example 'I noticed your doctor was talking to you for a long time. What did he have to say?'

Be aware of my own fears and pause before I say anything. Remind myself to talk less, when I am feeling nervous. Let the client speak first and lead the conversation.

To be more client-centred and follow the client's cues rather thinking about my own needs.

To listen and allow the client to talk.

Source: Adapted from Gibbs (1988)

The above model might be best suited for nurses new to the concept of reflective practice. As with all ongoing learning, nurses should demonstrate increased self-awareness, and greater depth and breadth of critical analysis, synthesis and evaluation. We will now briefly describe a more complex reflective model, which may be more appropriate for more senior learners and/or qualified staff.

Framework for reflective practice (Rolfe et al., 2001)

The What? model of reflection, by Rolfe et al. (2010), uses a questioning approach to facilitate the nurse to reflect on the three stages of the reflective process. The questions What? So what? and Now what? can stimulate reflection from novice to advanced levels. The model comprises three stages. Each stage has an extensive range of trigger questions, which aim to stimulate the mental health nurse's depth of thinking about the situation. The following illustrates a modified version of the What? model of reflection.

The What? model of reflection

Descriptive level of reflection	Understanding the context Theory and knowledge level of reflection	Action and future orientated level of reflection
What ... ↔ ↑ ... is the problem/difficulty/issue for feeling angry/not getting on /with client ... etc.? ... role did I have? ... actions did I take? ... did I hope to achieve? ... was my reaction to it? ... was the response of others? ... feeling did it evoke? ... in the patient? ... in myself? ... colleagues? ... was good/bad, useful/not useful about the experience?	**So what** ... ↔ ↑ ... does it tell me/mean to me about my client/our therapeutic relationship/my beliefs about mental health nursing/my role/my skills, etc.? ... did I base my actions on? ... was I thinking and feeling when I responded? ... other knowledge can I use to understand this event? ... could I have done differently?	**Now what** ... ↔ ↑ ... do I need to do differently to improve my skills/be more confident/be more effective/ get on better ... etc.? ... other issues do I need to consider for the future? ... might the consequences be if I do/don't do?

Source: Adapted from Rolfe et al. (2001)

Practice exercise

- Think of a recent interaction that took place during your clinical placement.
- When you have chosen your interaction, use the trigger questions described in Rolfe et al.'s model to reflect on your particular experience and the three stages of the reflective process.
- We would encourage you to keep brief notes about your thoughts, feelings and learning in your reflective journal and use them to discuss with your mentor or clinical supervisor.

Fostering reflection and reflective practice

A number of strategies are advocated to foster mental health nurses' reflective skills. These strategies aim to enhance the process of reflective learning and practice, and provide a sense of meaning for the mental health nurse, and are therefore an important component in the education of professionals (Biggs, 1999). As with any educational strategy, each reflective strategy presents different learning opportunities and challenges. We believe that having experience of the different strategies can provide a good learning opportunity for mental health nurses to develop their reflective ability and learning, both on their own and with and from others. For the mental health nurse, what is important is the ability to identify which strategy might best meet his/her learning needs at the different stages of their professional development. Strategies commonly used in practice include the following:

- reflective diaries/journals
- critical incidents based on practice
- reflective practice groups.

Reflective writing

The use of reflective writing is familiar to most nurses in the UK. Its value as a medium for developing reflective thinking skills and recording professional practice has received considerable attention in recent years. As an educational strategy, reflective writing is a potent and dynamic method for developing nurses' reflective ability and bridging the gap between theory and practice (Chirema, 2007). The reflective journal is regarded as an integral part of the student's professional and personal development. Mental health nurses are also encouraged to keep reflective journals post-registration as a means of supporting evidence for their continuing professional development (Nursing and Midwifery Council [NMC], 2002). The aim of a reflective journal is to enable the mental health nurse 'to learn from experiences throughout his/her professional life, by examining such experiences through regularly keeping a journal' (Sully and Dallas, 2005, p.23). However, the experience of journal keeping alone does not necessarily lead to learning. For learning to take place, the purpose of the reflective writing needs to be stated clearly and succinctly from the outset so that the focus is on the process and not the product (Craft, 2005). Furthermore, the issue(s) recorded in the journal must be made conscious, reflected on and lead to a change in understanding. The following are examples of reflective writing that focus on issues relating to Heron's communication framework, as written by Ali, a first-year mental health student.

Journal entries

Week 1: Date ...

'Today I was asked by a client what was Section 2 MHA (involuntary admission)? Providing information is what Heron calls an informative intervention. We learnt this in college but this was my first time to give information to a client. I knew what Section 2 was, so I felt OK telling the client this information. However, I wasn't sure if he understood all the points, he just said thanks and walked away. I felt at bit awkward and didn't say anything. In future, I need to sum up the key points and check if the client has understood what I said. I will talk about this with my mentor and find opportunities to practise it. Still it was a good experience, I enjoyed being able to provide the client with new information.'

Week 2: Date ...

'I observed my mentor carrying out an assessment today. It was very difficult; the client was depressed and spoke very slowly. My mentor was very good; she was so patient and allowed the client lots of time to speak. She also used a lot of open questions and paraphrasing, which helped to draw out the information from the client. My mentor told me she was using Heron's catalytic interventions. I was so glad I was just observing. I am impatient and I would have used closed questions. As a mental health nurse, I need to learn to slow things down and go at the client's pace when communicating. I also need to practise using open questions. I find it difficult not to use why questions. Hopefully, I will get better at this with practice.'

Week 3: Date ...

'Attended a case review meeting with my mentor. There were many different disciplines present including a doctor, social worker and psychologist. Each discipline talked about their area of work with the service user and her family. I learnt a lot about the different disciplines. I did not understand some of the things that they were talking about and I wanted to ask some questions, but I felt afraid that I would sound stupid. The staff nurse asked several questions. She spoke very confidently and was knowledgeable. I want to be like her when I qualify. After the meeting, she asked me about my impression of the meeting. This was very helpful; I felt she was genuinely interested in hearing my opinions. I wish other nurses did that. Instead they just tell you their opinion and are not interested in hearing different opinions, particularly a student's. It makes me feel very cross. I hope I don't do that when I qualify.'

Week 4: Date . . .

'Today was a really difficult day. I was talking to a client's mum. She visits her daughter Alicia every day, who was admitted last week following a serious suicide attempt. Her daughter is 21 years, the same age as me. Alicia's mum asked me when her daughter could go home. I told her that I didn't know but would ask the staff nurse and let her know. She thanked me and then started to cry. She kept apologizing for crying. I said to her it was OK. I felt so awkward. I know I am not good when people get upset. I need to learn how to use Heron's cathartic intervention.'

Week 5: Date . . .

'Had a really good day. I am really proud of myself. At the nursing handover I asked the staff nurse about her interventions with a specific client. She was a little taken aback, because I rarely speak in the handover. I was nervous when I spoke because there were at least five or more people at the handover and they were all more experienced than I am. However, I had thought about speaking at the handover quite a lot and I was determined to be more assertive, after all I had identified it as my goal since starting on the ward and that was over five weeks ago. Surprisingly, the staff nurse answered my question and was willing to teach me more about the use of CBT in clinical practice. I felt a bit embarrassed and uncomfortable as I had judged this nurse based on what other students said about her. I need to think about this in future and not allow myself to be influenced by others. I also need to be more assertive and ask questions. I can then learn so much more.'

Journal writing

In order to make the best use of journal writing and in accordance with good practice guidelines, it is important to pay attention to the following practices.

- Set time aside to write up your journal; where possible it is best to create a regular time/day for journal writing.

- Be creative, use diagrams, pictures and other sources to add to your reflections.
- Identify the purpose of your reflective writing at the beginning, for example you may wish to write about your use of a particular skill(s) such as open questions and listening during your placement.
- Write up your journal as soon as possible to enhance accuracy of recall.
- Ensure that the anonymity and confidentiality of persons/clients and institutions is protected by using no details that could identify individuals, contexts and/or situations. This is in keeping with the Nursing and Midwifery Council Code of Professional Conduct (NMC, 2002).
- Be mindful that the process of reflective writing can evoke different emotions, for example when writing and thinking about a client who has a long history of anorexia nervosa, the nurse became sad as she recalled painful memories of her own eating problems during adolescence.
- Seek support and guidance from your mentor, colleague or personal tutor to discuss any challenging issues that have arisen for you during your reflective writing.
- Be willing to use your reflective writing to share, discuss and learn with and from your colleagues and mentor in the clinical area.

The critical incident technique

The critical incident technique involves both writing about and reflecting on an experience or incident that occurred in the clinical setting. As an educational tool, it originated from Flanagan's (1954) work with WWII pilots as a means of classification and training method about effective or ineffective behaviour during aircraft combat missions. Since then, the critical incident technique has been used as a valuable educational tool in mental health nursing (Benson and Minghella, 1995). In itself, the critical incident provides a framework for reflection. A critical incident may include different types of clinical experiences, which are personal, unique and significant for the person, and may consist of an experience that:

- went unusually well
- did not go as planned
- is very ordinary and typical
- captures the essence of what nursing is all about
- was particularly demanding.

Reflection is the cornerstone of the critical incident technique and takes place when the student recalls the incident, identifies feelings, thoughts and behaviours, and in the analysis of the experience/incident makes inferences and evaluations, which in turn may illuminate future experiences (Ghaye and Lillyman, 1997). As such, it brings together practice and knowledge in mental health nursing and, as a result, the student may demonstrate learning outcomes from the experience within any of the educational domains – affective, cognitive or psychomotor skills. The following example illustrates a critical incident that occurred outside of the nurse's clinical practice and yet prompted significant learning for Louise, a third-year mental health student nurse.

Example of critical incident

Lucy, a third-year mental health student nurse, went to visit her elderly grandmother in hospital. She was very close to her grandmother and felt guilty that she had not visited her more often. On entering the ward, she saw her grandmother and waved. Her grandmother stared at her and then said, 'I do not know you, what do you want?' Lucy told her grandmother who she was, but her grandmother became quite distressed and kept shouting 'Go away; you are not my granddaughter.' Lucy felt upset and did not know what to do. Hearing raised voices, the staff nurse, Kate, approached Louise's grandmother and gently repeated 'it is OK Mrs White', until she became calmer. At the same time, Kate also suggested to Lucy that it might be best for her to wait outside for awhile.

When Mrs White was settled, Kate invited Lucy into a quiet room to discuss the recent incident. She listened attentively to Lucy as she talked about how upset she felt following her grandmother's response. Kate explained to Lucy that her grandmother's memory had deteriorated quite rapidly since her recent admission. Although still upset, Lucy appreciated the time, care and explanation she had received from Kate.

In the following days, Lucy thought a lot about this incident, in particular, the staff nurse's communication skills and her effective use of empathy, listening and information giving. Lucy reflected on her own communication skills and wondered whether she had responded in a similar manner when she encountered distressed family members and carers. Although she was now much more confident talking to families and carers, she recognized that she still found it uncomfortable when a family member or carer became upset. At such times, she often felt anxious and did not know what to say for fear of saying the wrong thing and upsetting the person further. Feeling a little embarrassed and uncomfortable about this new learning, she decided that she needed to discuss this with her mentor. She shared the incident and her learning with her mentor and discussed ways in which she could develop her communication skills, particularly when communicating with distressed families or carers.

Reflective practice groups

Another format commonly used in clinical practice to promote reflection comprises the reflective practice group. As an educational strategy, it provides the opportunity to share information, knowledge and experiences with others.

The reflective practice group usually takes place in the clinical setting whereby a senior or more experienced member of staff acts as a facilitator. As a teaching and learning strategy, the aim of the reflective practice group is to assist nurses to reflect on and examine their beliefs, actions and practice. For some nurses, having the opportunity to hear different perspectives to choose from can have a positive learning experience and enhance the mental health nurse's reflective skills (McGrath and Higgins, 2006). However, for others, sharing information about their clinical practice can be a threatening experience, often making them feel under scrutiny and anxious about being evaluated negatively by the facilitator and/or other members of the group. Essential to this experience is the facilitator's ability to assist the mental health nurse to overcome such fears.

The role of the reflective facilitator

Having a skilled and effective facilitator or mentor plays an important role in promoting reflective practice. The knowledge, skills and modelling that a facilitator conveys are important aspects of helping the mental health nurse to examine his/her thoughts, feelings and actions, and think deeply about their experience so that new learning can be acquired. Facilitators therefore need to be prepared and skilled in dealing with a wide range of professional and personal issues that might arise for student nurses in placement. However, not all good clinicians make good facilitators. Furthermore, each facilitator–learner relationship is different and is context-dependent. While there is a lack of empirical research in the nursing literature on what constitutes a good facilitator, the following characteristics have been identified as positive features for an effective facilitator (Fowler, 1995; Rolfe et al., 2010). These include the following:

- is approachable
- shows interest in learning
- demonstrates a willingness to facilitate learning in others while being open to learning about themselves
- is capable of forming a relaxed and supportive relationship
- has relevant knowledge and clinical skills
- can assess learning needs, facilitate reflection and evaluate learning
- is aware of the pressures and demands of students
- demonstrates effort in putting themselves out to help learners
- uses a wide range of teaching/learning methods that can be adapted to individual learners.

Organizational factors and reflection

The organizational setting and the hierarchical structure of the organization can influence the development of reflective practice and reflective practitioners. There may also be all sorts of pressures on either the learner or the qualified staff, or both, which may dictate whether reflective practice takes place. Such factors may include:

- staffing levels, for example there may be limited staff available and therefore time to foster reflective practice in the clinical setting
- organizational culture, for example if the clinical setting is not open or receptive to new ideas and/or examining or evaluating practice, then it is unlikely that reflective practice will occur
- nurses' educational experience, for example many registered nurses' training did not include or value the use of reflective practice.

Learning to become a reflective practitioner

The clinical setting provides a rich learning resource for both pre- and post-registered mental health nurses. However, experience alone is not the key to learning. Learning from experience in clinical practice involves reflection. While all of us have the potential to reflect, it is not an innate ability. Learning how to reflect on practice and develop the ability to become a more reflective practitioner requires time, commitment, and an open-mindedness to examine one's own practice, thoughts, feelings and responses. The process of reflection may at times be challenging and evoke feelings of discomfort and self-doubt. Nonetheless, engaging regularly in the process of reflection with your chosen reflective strategy and with the support of your mentor or others will assist you to gain confidence and learn from your increasing exposure to different and challenging experiences of mental health nursing. Learning to become a reflective practitioner is part of the nurse's ongoing professional and personal development. Reflection and reflective practice is part of a life long approach to learning.

Practice activity: reflecting on practice

The aim of this activity is to help you to monitor and develop your ability to become more reflective in your day-to-day practice as a mental health nurse.

Think back on the last week of your clinical placement and identify an interaction that you had with all of the following:

- service user
- family member/carer
- friend of service user.

Having identified the specific interactions, now answer the following questions. When you do so:

- be as truthful as you can and try not to censor your thoughts or feelings
- you may wish to write brief notes about your thoughts, feelings, observations, questions in your reflective journal and use them to discuss with your mentor

- it is important to note that some of the questions may prompt further questions, in such instances we encourage you to add or adapt the question(s) accordingly
- be mindful to take care of yourself; reflecting on specific experiences or events can evoke painful and uncomfortable feelings.

Questions for reflecting

1   What did you like about your communications/interactions with the service user, carer/family member or friend?
2   What did you *not* like about your communications/interactions with the service user, carer/family member or friend?
3   What skills do you currently hold?
4   Which of the interactions stands out for you and why?
5   Which interaction would you describe as your best and why?
6   Identify one thing that you have learnt from your interactions with the service user, carer/family member or friend?
7   If you could 'rewind' your interactions in practice, what would you do differently and why?
8   How do you know that your interactions with the service user, carer/family member or friend were effective?
9   Identify one communication skill or intervention that you want to develop/practise having reflected on your interactions.
10 Complete the following: if I were a service user, I would appreciate if nurses communicated more effectively by ... to me.
11 Complete the following: if I were a carer/family member, I would appreciate if nurses communicated more effectively by ... to me.
12 Complete the following: if I were a friend of the service user, I would appreciate if nurses communicated more effectively by ... to me.

Conclusion

There is little doubt that reflection and reflective practice play an important role for both pre- and post-registered mental health nurses' ongoing learning and development. However, reflection is a complex, demanding, life-long, purposeful activity. For the mental health nurse, it demands time, commitment and an openness to share and learn new ideas. As with most acquired skills, learning how to reflect takes time, practice and support from both nurse educators and nurse practitioners. Similar to other teaching and learning skills, it can be underused, undervalued and/or used ineffectively. Caution is therefore advised when implementing the use of reflective practice so that it enhances both the mental health nurse's ability to become a more reflective communicator. Although several studies provide support for the continuing use and development of reflective practice, there is a need for more empirical research to explain and support its effectiveness particularly in the area of mental health nursing.

Reflective questions

1　In your own words, how would you explain the concept of reflection?
2　What strategies or tools have you used to develop your ability to be more reflective, for example keeping a reflective diary, discussion with senior colleagues and how effective have they been in promoting your skills as a reflective practitioner?
3　What factors might encourage and/or discourage you from sharing your reflections with nursing colleagues in your practice area?
4　Reflecting on your current clinical placement, identify a communication issue(s) that you have reflected on. What have you learnt from this activity and how might you use this learning to develop your interpersonal skills in practice?

4 The therapeutic use of small talk: phatic communication

Introduction

Throughout this book, we examine how mental health nurses can communicate effectively with people in their care. We draw upon various therapeutic models of communication, counselling and therapy, and consider their application to the everyday therapeutic encounters that confront mental health nurses. Many of the chapters examine what might be called formal therapeutic approaches, guided by systematic application, and that often require further education and training in order for them to be practised safely, competently and efficiently. They also have a pre-determined and agreed end point.

However, many of the interactions mental health nurses have with service users are phatic communications – ordinary conversations that are free, aimless, social intercourse or (more commonly known as) small talk. These conversations seldom have a pre-determined outcome and involve nurses being with or attending to service users. They occur frequently and they can be found when studying the tasks that mental health nurses undertake in the course of their work, e.g. administering medication. While referred to as ordinary, studies of these conversations have increasingly shown them to be extraordinary, effective and appreciated by service users. We examine these encounters in this chapter. In particular, we consider:

- the concept of phatic communication
- its use and value in mental health nursing
- the evidence behind its use
- the link between phatic communication and brief ordinary and effective communication
- the application of these approaches in mental health nursing.

Learning outcomes

By the end of this chapter, you should be better able to:
1. Describe what is meant by phatic communication
2. Use phatic communication (small talk) effectively
3. Examine the concept of therapeutic use of self
4. Demonstrate the use of self in everyday communication

Phatic communication

Phatic communication is defined as 'ordinary chat or small talk' (Burnard 2003, p.678). The term 'phatic' (from the Greek *phatos*; speech) is from the same derivation as 'emphatic'. Emphatic communication usually has a pre-determined outcome and purpose, and is directed at the achievement of a specific result. The models of communication we address in Chapters 9, 10 and 11 are examples of emphatic approaches in which the content of the communication is central to whether it is effective or not. Phatic communication, on the other hand, focuses less on the content of communication, but more on the mere act of communicating. Examples of phatic communication are the everyday courtesies we extend to one another. When we greet someone with a 'Good morning, how are you?' we are simply acknowledging the person's presence, expressing politeness. To some degree it may be considered disingenuous when directed at strangers as more often than not we may not be that interested in how the person really is, but we are engaging in the sort of socially acceptable ritual that lies at the heart of civilized society. The value of phatic communication lies in recognizing its role in expressing camaraderie with the person to whom you are communicating. Phatic communication is generally taken at face value and a simple good morning directed at, or received from, another person makes both parties feel good. In other words, phatic communication is conversation for conversation's sake, as illustrated by the following examples.

Box 4.1 Examples of phatic communication

How are things?	Good morning
Nice day isn't it?	Nice to see you
Have a good day?	What's up?
Catch you later	It looks like rain today
Great weather we're having	The train must be running late

Phatic communication is common among many people, especially those that do not know one another, and is generally expected in routine conversation even among strangers. However, there some are dos and don'ts in using phatic communication and some of these are shown in Table 4.1. As we highlighted in Chapter 2, however, there are cultural differences in what may be acceptable and unacceptable topics of phatic communication. Be mindful of what may be culturally acceptable.

Using phatic communication in mental health nursing

Remember that the purpose of phatic communication is to establish social contact. As a mental health nurse, you might find phatic communication

Table 4.1 Dos and don'ts in using phatic communication

Do talk about	Don't talk about
The weather	Things that might cause offence
Current affairs	What a person earns
Sports	Personal issues, for example sexual practices
Entertainment	Controversial subjects, for example religion, politics
Things you have in common	Things that may be uncomfortable, for example
The prices in the shops	sensitive issues like weight

helpful as part of therapeutic engagement, but it may have limitations if it does not move beyond the point of initiating social contact, especially when the person is offering cues that not all may be well with them, as shown in the first practice exercise.

Practice exercise

Consider the following example of a phatic interaction that you might have with Mary, a service user with whom you are working.

Nurse: Good morning Mary, how are things?
Mary: Not too bad considering.
Nurse: Good, how are the children?
Mary: They're fine; I don't see them much as they're out most of the time.
Nurse: Just like mine, no time for me now that they think they're grown up.
Mary: Yes, I know what you mean.

This is a phatic conversation, but Mary has offered you a cue that things may not be so good and she wants to explore something that may be bothering her, but that you have overlooked. In other words, Mary appears to want the conversation to become emphatic. Re-write this brief script to detect the cue, act on it and turn the conversation emphatic.

Well, how did you do? Here's an example:

Nurse: Good morning Mary, how are things?
Mary: Not too bad considering.
Nurse: Considering? That does not sound so good.
Mary: Well, I've been hearing voices that are troubling me again.
Nurse: OK, tell me exactly how troubling they are.
Mary: I feel that I want to harm myself.
Nurse: OK, let's think about how we'll deal with this.

Table 4.2 Possibilities and pitfalls in phatic conversations

Possibilities	Pitfalls
Helps work with uncomfortable silences	Could miss cues that require therapeutic intervention
Demonstrates spontaneity	
Intuitive, e.g. done without much thought	Listener may get impatient
Uses own experience	Danger of undermining professional credibility
Not impeded by issues of confidentiality	Inclination to compete to take turns
Not forced	Danger that you may be communicating insignificance
Relies on little formal skill	
Does not need costly training or preparation	Speech could appear ritualized, conventional and pedestrian
Not bound by formal rules of communication	
Breaks down professional barriers	Not essential to development of sound interpersonal skills

In the second example, you have picked up the cue from Mary and acted upon it, thereby turning the conversation into an emphatic one. Had you continued with the phatic conversation it may have derailed the interaction.

The emphatic conversation shown in the second example illustrates the difference between a professional helping relationship that you have with a service user, and the phatic nature of a personal helping relationship that you may have with a friend. Your relationship with service users as a mental health nurse is a professional helping one in which you practise your art, craft and science with a particular purpose. However, in the course of a typical working day, you are likely to have many phatic encounters. In Table 4.2, we outline the possibilities and pitfalls of phatic conversations.

In Chapter 2, Figure 2.1, we demonstrated the skills mental health nurses use when talking with acutely psychotic people; one of these was 'being with the patient' (Bowers et al., 2009). Part of being with the patient is light, casual, normal conversation and this is similar to phatic communication.

Practice exercise

Consider the sort of encounters that you have in your day-to-work work. Make a list of those times when you used phatic conversations.

- What were those conversations?
- When did they occur?
- Why did they occur?
- What followed them?
- Who initiated them?
- What was the outcome?

So far, in this chapter we have described phatic communication and how mental health nurses can use it in their day-to-day work. In the next section, we examine the model of brief, ordinary and effective communication (Crawford et al., 2006).

Brief, ordinary and effective (BOE) communication

BOE communication is rooted in the work of Alvin Toffler, who, in 1980, predicted a future where we would be exposed to short blips of intensive information usually in the form of adverts, sound bites, and snippets of news like the 60-second news updates commonly seen between many longer news bulletins on television today. While there are attempts to reverse this culture among many groups, to a large degree Toffler's predictions 30 years ago are now commonplace and are more or less subsumed into modern society. The use of texts and the development of social networking sites such as Facebook and Twitter are examples of the use of the sort of blips to which Toffler refers.

In this book, we argue for the importance of effective communication in the provision of safe, sound and secure mental health nursing. We describe many types of communication. Some of these, e.g. solution-focused interventions (see Chapter 10), require additional training if they are to be practised safely and effectively; in other words they require time. However, time is increasingly in short supply in many health and social care settings. Surveys of mental health service users, such as the national patient surveys that the Care Quality Commission in England (CQC) conduct on an annual basis (see CQC, 2009, for example), report consistently that therapeutic time is something service users value, but that mental health professionals seldom have.

Whilst recognizing the importance of providing time for mental health nurses to care, time is a necessary, but insufficient condition for care to thrive. If mental health nurses are to provide effective care through sound interpersonal skills, they will need to use their time well. Even when mental health nurses have time to care, care does not always result. Providing therapeutic care through effective communication requires mental health nurses to apply, what is commonly referred to as the emotional labour of nursing. The emotional labour of mental health nursing may cause nurses high levels of stress (Mann and Cowburn, 2005). Therefore, mental health nurses may be avoiding therapeutic contact with service users as a means of minimizing emotional labour and protecting themselves from unwanted stress.

Examples of emotional labour are:

- consistently showing compassion
- having lots of therapeutic encounters
- high levels of intensity in each encounter

- highly expressed emotions (for example, anger, distress) by service users or their significant others
- the discussion of highly sensitive issues.

Practice exercise

Think of therapeutic encounters that you have experienced with service users lately. These encounters may have taken place at various locations. Describe one such encounter and reflect on what was the emotional work that this required. How did you deal with this emotional work?

BOE communication acknowledges the time constraints under which many healthcare professionals work. It recognizes the emotional work tied into many therapeutic encounters. The BOE model is an attempt to address the lack of time and the emotional work of mental health nursing. It is underpinned by an understanding that:

- phatic communication is common in health care encounters
- patients do not often want prolonged encounters
- brief encounters can leave a mark on people – the epiphany moment
- ordinary encounters may mask more complex styles of communication.

The characteristics of the BOE model are shown in Table 4.3.

Crawford et al. (2006) identify 31 core skills considered central to BOE communication. The skills proposed incorporate aspects of effective communication that we address in this book. In Table 4.4, we reproduce these skills.

Table 4.3 Characteristics of the brief, ordinary and effective model of communication (Brown et al., 2006; Crawford et al., 2006)

Brief	Ordinary	Effective
Brief communications can create and maintain a therapeutic alliance Mental health nurses can exploit tasks, such as administering medication, to communicate effectively Using such tasks can help mental health nurses demonstrate sound interpersonal skills by listening actively, communicating genuineness, warmth and empathy	People value and are comfortable with ordinary conversations Ordinary conversations equalize the encounter Ordinary conversations minimize the likelihood of nurses using jargon to distance themselves from service users Ordinary conversations allow service users to share their stories in a non-threatening manner.	Linked to positive clinical outcomes Values, culture and evidence-based Service users are satisfied Can be captured, audited and evaluated

Table 4.4 Core skills in brief, ordinary and effective communication (Brown et al., 2006; Crawford et al., 2006). Reproduced with the permission of Nelson Thornes Ltd from Communications in Clinical Settings, Crawford et al, 978-0-7487-9716-5, first published in 2006.

BOE core skills

1. Making oneself approachable and available to service users, their carers or relatives, colleagues and partners from other statutory and non-statutory services
2. Demonstrating basic interpersonal skills in terms of appropriate eye contact, posture, proximity, relaxed manner, touch
3. Welcoming and initiating friendly and appropriate conversation
4. Conducting and sustaining polite, balanced, shared conversation with appropriate turn-taking and use of non-verbal and verbal prompts, i.e. head nods and hand gestures; phrases such as 'go on', 'I see', 'OK', and expressions such as 'uh-huh'
5. Ending or closing conversation in a mutually satisfying and respectful manner
6. Creating and sustaining rapport with others through active listening, attending, reflecting feelings, warmth, empathy, genuineness, being non-judgemental and accepting
7. Frequently acknowledging others by using brief, positive greetings, ordinary/everyday conversation, or by engaging non-verbally, for example through eye contact, smiling and nodding
8. Using empowering language that encourages self-determination and decision-making of others
9. Using non-stigmatizing language – avoiding the use of labels or descriptions that isolate, belittle or are abusive to others
10. Using dignified or self-respecting language
11. Negotiating care with service users in the spirit of concordance (reaching agreement)
12. Using simple activities to promote relationships with service users, such as bed-making, helping with meals, making a drink, washing or mobilizing, etc.
13. Demonstrating appropriate use of silence, for example in facilitating reflection, expression of feelings, conveying empathy; to encourage response to open questions; as an opportunity to observe or convey interest
14. Demonstrating appropriate use of humour to create an open, responsive social atmosphere; relax others and reduce stress; reach out to and engage others; increase interaction; and boost morale
15. Demonstrating a willingness simply to be in the presence of service users
16. Giving feedback to others that is constructive and facilitates positive change
17. Receiving and giving appropriate consideration to feedback from service users, carers, relatives and colleagues
18. Accurately interpreting and confirming (under supervision) non-verbal communication from service users, carers, relatives and colleagues
19. Using appropriate open or closed questioning, being aware that asking too many questions may be stressful
20. Responding to questions in an honest and clear manner
21. Clarifying or checking out the meaning of what people say by careful use of questioning, summarizing and paraphrasing; this is especially important when dealing with complex issues

(continued)

Table **4.4** Core skills in brief, ordinary and effective communication (Brown et al., 2006; Crawford et al., 2006). Reproduced with the permission of Nelson Thornes Ltd from Communications in Clinical Settings, Crawford et al, 978-0-7487-9716-5, first published in 2006. (*continued*)

BOE core skills

22. Demonstrating sensitivity to the communication needs of people when English is their second language
23. Brief, time-limited counselling applied to specific service user situations (under supervision)
24. Communicating appropriately with individuals who have visual, hearing, speech or cognitive disabilities.
25. Identifying anxiety, depression and confusion, and how these may affect communication ability
26. Identifying anger and frustration, and using verbal and non-verbal de-escalation techniques
27. Providing sensitive, emotional support to colleagues and team members
28. Providing accurate advice, instruction, information and professional opinion to service users, carers, relatives and colleagues; and when necessary to groups of colleagues or service users/carers/relatives
29. Maintaining confidentiality in both spoken and written communication
30. Answering telephone enquiries in an appropriate manner: identifying oneself, being polite, striving to reduce hostility or conflict, resolving queries or concerns
31. Keeping brief, factual and accurate care records

Practice exercise

Consider the core skills of BOE shown in Table 4.4. In Table 2.3 we described the five key components of developing, maintaining and ending therapeutic encounters. These are:

- core attitudes and values
- setting clinical boundaries
- developing the encounter
- maintaining the encounter
- ending the encounter.

Now consider the core skills of BOE shown in Table 4.4. Place each of the core skills into one of the five key components of developing, sustaining and ending therapeutic encounters.

The application of BOE in mental health nursing

Having linked the core skills of BOE to the five categories of therapeutic communication, we now want you to assess yourself against these core skills. Using a SWOT analysis, we want you to identify those skills where you have

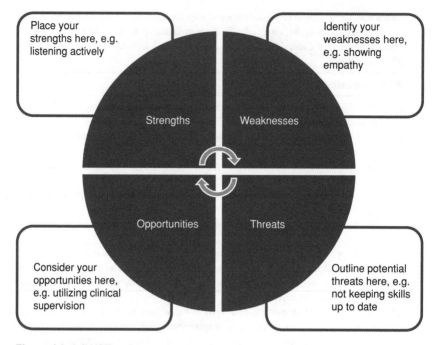

Figure 4.1 A SWOT analysis to assess core skills in BOE

Strengths and Weaknesses, those that provide Opportunities to improve your communication skills and those that may Threaten your attempts to practise effective communication. You can copy the diagram in Figure 4.1 to help you in this exercise.

Having considered phatic communication and examined the BOE model of communication, we now consider the concept of therapeutic use of self.

Therapeutic use of self

Therapeutic use of self occurs when health professionals consciously use their 'personality, insights, perceptions, and judgements as part of the therapeutic process' (Punwar and Peloquin, 2000, p.285). In Chapter 2, we reported on the evidence for what works for whom in psychotherapeutic exchanges and showed consistently that many factors independent of any therapeutic model were more strongly linked to positive outcomes. It is these factors that we call the 'therapeutic use of self'. There are several components of the therapeutic use of self:

- personality, insights, perceptions and judgements
- self-awareness
- self-concept

- self-esteem
- self-efficacy
- self-confidence.

We will now describe each of these components and show how to use them in therapeutic communication.

Personality factors

- A high degree of self-confidence, e.g. taking risks
- Being open and honest about your skills
- Flexibility, for example trying out new ideas
- Expressing humility, for example accepting that you may not have all the answers

Insight is largely concerned with a high degree of self-awareness. Perceptions and judgements include insight, but also recognizing the individuality of the client, using self-disclosure and, expressing empathy, and person-centred skills such as unconditional positive regard. Although these factors are often regarded as model independent, they are more closely associated with person-centred, humanistic approaches.

Self-awareness

The use of self, a core issue in therapeutic use of self, has many dimensions and we shall consider some of these. The first is self-awareness; a mental health nurse using himself/herself therapeutically is likely to be self-aware. To be self-aware means:

- reflecting upon ourselves
- paying attention to ourselves
- identifying what it is within ourselves that we can use therapeutically.

Reflection is an important part of being self-aware. The use of a reflective model described in Chapter 3 may help this process.

Self-concept

Self-concept is another dimension of using oneself therapeutically. Self-concept is about expressing one's true self, or as Rowan (2001), a humanistic therapist, calls it, the authentic self. In expressing your authentic self in your mental health nursing, you are likely to express those aspects of yourself that reflect your humanity. When you act selflessly in carrying out your role as a mental health nurse you recognize the requirement to put the interests of the patient above your own and the patient has a sense of you acting sincerely (authentically). An example of this is expressing 'genuineness'. Genuineness stems from the work of Carl Rogers's person-centred therapy (Rogers, 1961). A mental health nurse who is genuine will act in manner congruent with how he/she feels. For example, what you say is matched by how you behave, nodding your head when verbally expressing agreement. We call this verbal/non-verbal congruity.

Practice exercise

Consider the concept of genuineness shown above. Think about your practice and write down specific examples of occasions when you have expressed genuineness.

Self-esteem

Self-esteem is an assessment of your self-worth and includes beliefs about yourself, such as 'I am good at communicating empathy', and the expression of emotions such as hope, despair and pride. A high level of self-esteem is thought necessary to using yourself therapeutically; if you believe yourself capable and competent, and can convey this to others in a professional helping relationship, you can be more therapeutic. You can assess your level of self-esteem using a standard questionnaire such the Rosenberg Self-Esteem Scale (Rosenberg, 1965).

1 Overall, I am satisfied with myself.
2 At times, I think that I am no good at all.
3 I feel that I have a number of good qualities.
4 I am able to do things as well as most other people.
5 I feel I do not have much to be proud of.
6 I certainly feel useless at times.
7 I feel that I am a person of worth, at least the equal of others.
8 I wish I could have more respect for myself.
9 Overall, I am inclined to feel that I am a failure.
10 I take a positive attitude towards myself.

You answer each statement (item) by stating your level of agreement from strongly agree, agree, disagree or strongly disagree.

For statements 1, 3, 4, 7 and 10 strongly agree scores 4, agree scores 3, disagree scores 2 and strongly disagree scores 1.

However, for items 2, 5, 6, 8 and 9 the scores are reversed, i.e. for these items strongly agree scores 1, agree scores 2, disagree scores 3 and strongly disagree scores 4.

Once you have answered each statement you add up all your scores to each and this gives you a total score. For example, if you answer strongly agree to items 1, 3, 4, 7 and 10, and strongly disagree to items 2, 5, 6, 8 and 9, your total score will be 40 indicating the highest level of self-esteem.

A score of 20 suggests a moderate level of self-esteem and scores below this indicate a low level of self-esteem.

Practice exercise

We want you to rate your level of self-esteem using the scale above. Look at each statement carefully and answer: strongly agree, agree, disagree or strongly disagree to each one. Now calculate your self-esteem score using the scoring system shown above. Now reflect on your level of self-esteem. Is it high, moderate or low? How do you think your level of self-esteem affects your ability to use yourself therapeutically?

Self-efficacy

To show self-efficacy is to show belief in your confidence to change your behaviour from an unhealthy to a healthier one and derives from the work of the psychologist Albert Bandura in 1997 and his Social Cognitive Theory of learning and behaving. In general, the higher your level of self-efficacy, the better your performance. Low levels of self-efficacy are likely to reduce your performance. There are four main sources of self-efficacy.

1 **Mastery** is a situation whereby you have developed expertise in some skill; it is usually demonstrated by regular success when using this skill. This success raises self-efficacy. Mastery usually results from education and training, repeated practice and feedback on performance. For example, it is hoped that by reading this book and working through the practice exercises and reflective questions, and applying these skills in your everyday practice, you will develop mastery in fundamental communication skills.

2 **Modelling** is where you demonstrate (model) your communication skills and the successful outcome of these skills, to others so that they can learn from you. Modelling is not always intentional; people with less experience than you may be watching how you work from a distance and picking up tips on what may happen if they model your behaviour. Modelling works better when the person is a peer.

3 **Social persuasion** is feedback from others. This feedback can be positive, i.e. encouraging, or negative, i.e. discouraging. Positive feedback is likely to increase your level of self-efficacy, whereas negative feedback is likely to lower your self-efficacy. The feedback must feel genuine, i.e. the person to whom it is given must value it and feel that it is given authentically.

4 **Physiological features** are the body's responses to external stimuli. For example, stress is a physiological response. Physiological responses can affect self-efficacy in several ways. If you feel stressed before seeing a client and you are low in self-efficacy you are likely to perceive this stress as an example of how poor you are at communicating with clients. If your self-efficacy level is high, you are likely to perceive the stress as a sign of how interested, skilled and ready you are to be therapeutic.

In Chapter 11, we discuss the role of self-efficacy in motivational interviewing.

Self-confidence

Self-confidence is a belief in your confidence that you can be therapeutic. If you are self-confident, you are likely to find being therapeutic less of a challenge and you are more able to use yourself therapeutically. Examples of being self-confident are:

- you can identify easily many qualities about yourself
- when you are in the presence of others you can hold your own
- you make friends easily
- you can express an opinion assertively even in the face of strong disagreement from others
- you can easily overcome difficulties.

You can test your self-confidence levels by checking how you would answer questions such as:

- How much do you trust decisions that you take?
- How worried would you be if you were asked to make a presentation to colleagues?
- How would you feel if you were to disagree with your boss?
- How helpless would you feel if a service user resisted any attempts to help her/him?
- How likely is it that you would volunteer to run a therapeutic group on your own?

If you trust decisions that you make, are not worried about giving a presentation to colleagues, feel able to disagree with your boss, are able to deal with service users' resistance and would have little problem running a therapeutic group on your own, you are high in self-confidence. If you are uncomfortable with doing these things, you are low in self-confidence. If this is the case, here are some ways in which you can improve your self-confidence, by:

- speaking assertively, for example 'I disagree with your views'
- identifying your contribution to your team's successes
- staying in shape physically, for example exercising regularly
- expressing your view even if it is unpopular
- speaking clearly and with little hesitation
- being prepared to praise others for their achievements even if this has meant disappointment for you.

Practice exercise

Identify three therapeutic encounters you have had recently. Identify examples from these encounters when you have demonstrated the therapeutic use of self. What aspect of the self did you demonstrate? How did you use it? How did the patient respond? What was the outcome of each encounter? What part, if any, did you feel that using yourself therapeutically played in the outcome of each encounter?

In summary, the therapeutic use of self requires you to reflect on what personal qualities, as opposed to skills, you bring to the therapeutic encounter. To use yourself therapeutically, it is thought important to be open, self-aware, have a strong self-concept, and exhibit high levels of self-esteem and self-confidence. These qualities appear independent of whatever model of therapeutic intervention you may be using. The final part of this chapter will consider evidence for the efficacy and effectiveness of small talk in communication.

The efficacy and effectiveness of small talk

To our best knowledge, there has been little systematic investigation of the efficacy and effectiveness of phatic communication in mental health nursing. However, there is inferred evidence that has a long history dating back to the cultural anthropologist Bronislaw Malinowski's original studies of the Argonauts of the South Pacific where phatic communication appeared to foster everyday interaction. In Table 4.2, we show some of the pitfalls of phatic communication. Arguably, phatic communication provides an opportunity to initiate a therapeutic encounter, but it is not clear whether it is an added extra or essential to the therapeutic encounter being established.

The evidence for the BOE model derives from the effectiveness outcomes that Crawford et al. (2006) and Brown et al. (2006) report; examples of these are shown in Table 4.3. It is not clear, however, what clinical outcomes the use of BOE communication might generate specifically, or whether these outcomes might have resulted simultaneously. The core skills of BOE shown in Table 4.4 include examples of verbal and non-verbal communication skills that have a fairly well-established evidence base. Many of the core skills shown in Table 4.4, however, appear to require more than brief interventions, mixed with those that could be applied in brief encounters. The model appears less parsimonious as a result.

The therapeutic use of self has been studied quite extensively and, when the contents are unpacked, there is a fairly strong evidence base for the role of therapist-orientated factors. From this evidence, it is clear that mental health nurses have the necessary opportunities to use themselves therapeutically, and in many respects can use these opportunities with minimal additional education or training. Clinical supervision may be an important prerequisite for using oneself therapeutically.

Conclusion

An often overlooked aspect of effective communication is the use of phatic conversations, brief, ordinary and effective communications, and the therapeutic use of self. Mental health nurses are well placed to take advantage of these approaches to enhance their communication skills in everyday clinical encounters. These skills can be used whatever the clinical encounter, whether it is task-based or part of a one-to-one pre-planned interaction with another person.

Reflective questions

1   What are the advantages and disadvantages of using phatic communication in everyday social interactions?
2   How can you use phatic communication in your work as a mental health nurse? Give specific examples.
3   How many core skills in BOE communication can you identify? Write these down.
4   Why might you use yourself therapeutically in mental health nursing?

5 Heron's communication framework: Six Category Intervention Analysis

Introduction

Communication is a fundamental component of all therapeutic interventions and is essential for the delivery of quality nursing care. Mental health practice needs nurses who can offer more skilled and effective therapeutic communication (Department of Health (DH), 2006). Acquiring new skills that are therapeutic, and learning how to use them effectively should help to improve mental health nurses' knowledge and skill base, so that they can provide best practice in a variety of clinical situations. In mental health nursing several different models of communication are taught and applied in clinical practice, for example Egan's model of helping, cognitive behaviour therapy (CBT) and solution-focused approach. The latter therapeutic approaches are currently receiving increasing popularity in nurse education and clinical practice. These will be addressed later in the book. For this chapter, we have chosen Heron's (2001) Six Category Intervention Analysis model of communication. As a communication model, we believe it not only provides a flexible, user friendly framework to develop nurses' therapeutic interventions, but also facilitates the application of communication skills in in various clinical encounters. In addition, this model can be used by learners at different levels of their professional and personal learning and in varied clinical situations.

Learning outcomes

By the end of this chapter, you should be better able to:

1 Describe Heron's Six Category Intervention Analysis model
2 Demonstrate an understanding of how each of the six interventions can be used in clinical practice
3 Use Heron's six categories in clinical practice

The Six Category Intervention Analysis

John Heron's Six Category model is a well-known communication/counselling framework, which was originally published in 1975, by the Human Potential Research Project at the University of Surrey (Heron, 1975). Since then, it has been revised, expanded and used as the basis of interpersonal training, with a wide range of professions, including mental health nursing (Heron, 1977, 1996, 1999, 2001). As a therapeutic model, it presents six different forms of helping behaviour also known as categories, which can be used when working face-to-face with a client, their family or others involved in their care. Each of the six categories and the respective interventions that fall under each category are *theoretically neutral* – that is, they are not aligned with any particular theoretical perspective, for example a humanistic approach, cognitive behavioural therapy and others (Heron, 2001). This means that Heron's Six Category model can be used either on its own or along with another therapeutic approach used in mental health practice. Similar to other psychotherapeutic approaches, the quality of the nurse–client relationship is paramount to the therapeutic use and outcome of each of the six categories.

As a communication model, the Six Category framework:

- offers a relationship that is grounded in a client-centred attitude
- provides a tool for the mental health nurse to monitor, select and review his/her communication skills and interactions
- identifies a repertoire of interventions that can be used in a wide range of communication encounters, whereby the mental health nurse is the *listener* and the client the *talker* and the person who is dealing with some issue, that needs the time, attention and service of another human being
- classifies a huge range of communication skills under six categories, which are six kinds of purpose or intention.

Authoritative and facilitative interventions

The six forms of helping behaviour are classified into two main groups: authoritative and facilitative interventions.

Authoritative interventions	Facilitative interventions
Authoritative interventions are so called because:	**Facilitative** interventions are so called because:
• the mental health nurse is taking a more directive role and is taking more responsibility for or on behalf of the client • the emphasis is more on what the mental health nurse is doing to the client • authoritative interventions include: prescriptive; informative; confronting	• the role of the mental health nurse is less hierarchical • the mental health nurse's interventions try to enable the client to become more autonomous and take on more responsibility for themselves • facilitative interventions include: catalytic; cathartic; supportive

Authoritative and facilitative categories

Authorative	Faciliatative
Prescriptive	Catalytic
Informative	Cathartic
Confronting	Supportive

Source: Heron (2001)

Interventions and intention

The Six Category model comprises six types of intervention that the practitioner or mental health nurse can use as part of his/her work with the client. 'An intervention is an identifiable piece of verbal and/or non verbal behaviour that is part of the practitioner's service to the client' (Heron, 2001, p.3). There is, however, no set or prescribed verbal formula for stating an intervention. An intervention can consist of many variations of verbal and non-verbal formats, all of which are dependent on the context of the interaction, and the nature of the relationship between the client and the mental health nurse. While the six interventions refer mostly to the nurse's verbal skills, components of non-verbal behaviour, for example eye contact, gestures and other non-verbal behaviours, are equally important in determining how the verbal interventions come across to the client. The mental health nurse therefore needs to be mindful about not only what s/he says, but also how it is expressed. It is also important that verbal and non-verbal messages are congruent – that is, what is being said is also reflected by the body language that is being conveyed. The following examples illustrate a range of verbal interventions, which are commonly used by mental health nurses in clinical practice.

Verbal interventions used in mental health practice

- 'When you feel a panic attack, I want you to take a deep breath and count to 10'
- 'I want you to sit here and tell me what prompted you to break the window'
- 'Sleep disturbance is a symptom of depression'
- 'The drug you are taking does increase your appetite'
- 'I am disappointed that you did not cancel your appointment'
- 'It seems that what you say and what you do mean different things'
- 'When did you start to feel depressed?'
- 'What prompted you to cut yourself?'
- 'It's OK to feel angry'
- 'It's OK to cry'

(continued)

- 'I know that wasn't easy for you, but I am pleased that you were able to say no'
- 'It must be hard for you as a parent seeing your son so distressed, yet you are always so positive and encouraging to him'

Intention

All six categories comprise a specific intention or purpose that determines the choice of intervention. Each intervention can be defined in terms of its intention or purpose – that is, what it is that the mental health nurse wants to achieve by his/her intervention. The following outlines the six categories and the primary intention behind each intervention (Heron, 2001). Examples of the different categories commonly used by mental health nurses are also illustrated.

Six categories and their intentions

Category: Prescriptive

Intention: a prescriptive intervention aims to direct the behaviour of the client by demonstration, advice, suggestion, command, propose, order, insist.

Examples

- 'Show me what medication you take'
- 'I want you to attend the anxiety management group'
- 'I think you might feel better if you have a bath'
- 'I want you to tell me when you feel the urge to cut yourself'
- 'Do the following breathing exercises every time you feel panicky'
- 'Listen to your music, that might help to "tune out" the voices'
- 'I want you to leave the ward now'
- 'You need to drink a litre of fluids a day for the next two days because you are dehydrated'
- 'I think this might be a good time to discuss how you feel about being discharged to the hostel'
- 'You need to contact the social worker about your son's accommodation'

Category: Informative

Intention: an informative intervention aims to impart new knowledge/information to the client by telling, informing, lecturing and using one's expertise.

Examples

- 'One of the side effects of your medication is constipation'
- 'Anxiety can cause you to have palpitations'
- 'There is a support group for carers every Monday'
- 'Section 2 of the Mental Health Act is for 28 days'
- 'This is the information I promised about WRAP, which stands for Wellness Recovery Action Plan'
- 'CBT stands for cognitive behaviour therapy'
- 'In my experience, distraction techniques are a useful strategy to manage anxiety'
- 'ECT stands for electro-convulsive therapy'
- 'Maintaining social contacts and finding suitable activities or work is important for a person's mental wellbeing and recovery'
- 'MIND is an important mental health charity and provides useful information'

Category: Confronting

Intention: a confronting intervention aims to raise the consciousness (awareness) of the client about some limiting attitude, belief or behaviour that he or she is unaware of by challenging, and giving direct feedback in a supportive manner.

Examples

- 'I am aware that you have not attended the day centre for the past two weeks'
- 'I have noticed that you find it difficult to ask for help'
- 'Are you aware that your son has made a serious suicide attempt?'
- 'I have noticed that you never talk about the positive things in your life'
- 'I was disappointed that you didn't phone to cancel our appointment yesterday'
- 'You say *no one* cares for you, yet your family visit every day?'
- 'Are you aware that you tend to interrupt others when they are talking?'
- 'You ask to speak to me and yet when I try to talk to you, you avoid me'
- 'Your son is trying very hard to manage his voices and live an independent life. I notice that you tend to focus on the things that he does not do well as opposed to the things that he does do well'
- 'Are you aware that your mother feels frightened when you start shouting?'

Category: Catalytic

Intention: a catalytic intervention aims to enable the client to learn and develop by self-direction, problem solving and self-discovery within the context of the nurse – client encounter, but also beyond it.

(continued)

Examples

- 'What helps you to cope with the voices?'
- 'What is your understanding of schizophrenia?'
- 'Say more about what you think of when you want to harm yourself'
- 'What was it like being admitted to the mental health unit?'
- 'Tell me more about the things that keep you well'
- 'When you feel depressed, what do you think about?'
- 'How does the rest of the family manage when your son is unwell?'
- 'Which problem would you like to look at today?'
- 'What can I do to help you?'
- 'What do you want from your family?'

Category: Cathartic

Intention: a cathartic intervention aims to enable the client to share, express or discharge painful emotions – primarily grief, fear and anger – by encouraging and supporting the person to express his/her feelings.

Examples

- 'I imagine you must feel very frightened being in hospital for the first time?'
- 'You seem very upset; it is OK to feel sad'
- 'Will you say that again, louder ... louder?'
- 'You said you felt so angry towards your father, would you like to talk about it?'
- 'It's OK to cry'
- 'Feeling angry is normal'
- 'Some people find that writing a letter can help to release emotions'
- 'I notice you are tearful when you talk about your dad. It must be difficult for you when he says, I don't know you'
- 'It's OK to feel sad and grieve for your brother'
- 'It's OK to feel anxious about your father's prognosis'

Category: Supportive

Intention: a supportive intervention aims to affirm the worth and value of the client's qualities, attitudes or actions by enhancing the self-esteem of the person by giving encouraging feedback and validating.

Examples

- 'You have done your best to help your daughter'
- 'You made a great effort to participate in the group'
- 'I think you did everything you could to keep your son at home'
- 'I appreciate you being honest with me and telling me how you really feel'

- 'I admire your determination to stay sober'
- 'I know that asking for help is a big step for you'
- 'You managed your anger very effectively in the meeting'
- 'I really admire your positive attitude in spite of all the difficulties you have faced'
- 'Well done for stating your needs in the group'
- 'I admire your courage to be open with your family and friends about your experiences of being in hospital for mental health problems'

Source: Heron (2001)

Applying Six Category Intervention Analysis

When using the different interventions in clinical practice, it is important to remember that the authoritative categories are 'neither more nor less valuable or useful' than the facilitative interventions (Heron, 2001, p.6). Similarly, each of the six interventions is *value neutral* – that is, each intervention is equally important and valuable when used in the appropriate context. The choice of intervention will depend on the:

- nature of the nurse's role at the time
- particular needs of the client
- content or focus of the intervention.

In practice, however, authoritative interventions have traditionally tended to be overused. Studies of qualified nurses' perception of their interpersonal skills using Six Category Intervention Analysis found that nurses generally perceived themselves to be more skilful in the authoritative categories (Burnard and Morrison, 1988, 1989, 1991). A decade later, participants attending Six Category training workshops identified confronting and cathartic interventions as their least skilled categories (Heron, 2001). While authoritative interventions are valuable and at times necessary, they can become ineffective and therefore non-therapeutic when they are over-used, and/or used to the exclusion of facilitative interventions. Equally, it is inappropriate to use facilitative interventions exclusively, particularly if such interventions prohibit the use of the nurse's authority in an appropriate and professional way. For example, in practice there may be occasions when it is part of mental health nurses' role and responsibility to use prescriptive, informative and/or confronting interventions at a particular time, as illustrated by the following examples:

- Prescriptive – 'I would like you to take your medication'
- Prescriptive – 'I want you to stay on the ward for now'
- Prescriptive – 'I will remove the sharp objects from your bag, they will be returned to you when you are discharged'

- Informative – 'One of the side effects of your medication is low blood pressure'
- Informative – 'ECT stands for electro-convulsive therapy'
- Informative – 'Sleep disturbance is a symptom of depression'
- Confronting – 'It sounds like you were asked to leave the hostel because you were aggressive towards the other residents'
- Confronting – 'Are you aware that you frighten other clients when you start shouting?'
- Confronting – 'I notice that you find it difficult to ask for help'

In practice, balancing authoritative and facilitative interventions is about the appropriate use of power between the client and the mental health nurse (Heron, 2001) and includes the following forms of power:

- the mental health nurse's power over the client, for example the nurse's power in his/her capacity as a mental health professional
- the power shared between the mental health nurse and the client, for example, the nurse and client's power to ask questions and to listen to each other
- the autonomous power within the client, for example the client's power to make decisions about his/her life.

The above forms of power are interrelated, and will change according to the changing needs of the client throughout the therapeutic relationship. The following clinical scenario illustrates an interaction whereby the mental health nurse uses authoritative and facilitative interventions.

Clinical scenario

Adam, a third-year student, enjoys working in the Day Hospital for the Older Adult. He has a good relationship with the clients, their families and carers. The staff nurse asked Adam to inform Mrs Black about the carers' support group. Mrs Black has cared for her husband who has short-term memory impairment for over five years. They have no children. Mr Black attends the Day Hospital three days a week. The following illustrates the interaction that took place.

Adam: 'How are you today?' [Catalytic]

Mrs Black: 'Fine thank you. I am so looking forward to my holiday in a few weeks. I need a rest, I am so tired.'

Adam: 'I am sorry to hear that. I thought you looked tired. What's causing you to be so tired?' [Supportive and Catalytic]

Mrs Black: 'Oh it's nothing; I just need a good rest.'

Adam: 'How is your sleep these days?' [Catalytic]

Mrs Black: 'It's OK.'

Adam: 'OK?' [Catalytic]

Mrs Black: 'Oh I get a few hours.'

Adam: 'Mrs Black, I might be wrong but I sense that you are not telling me something?' [Confronting]

Mrs Black: [Starting to cry] 'I am sorry I know you want to help but I am afraid to tell you what's been happening as you will think I can't cope.'

Adam: 'From what I know of you, I think you cope very well caring for your husband.' [Supportive]

Mrs Black: 'My husband is waking up every night and wandering around the house, saying he wants to go to work. He only sleeps for three or four hours. I don't know what to do, I have tried everything.'

Adam: 'That must be very difficult for you. It is so important that you and your husband get adequate sleep. I think you should see the clinical nurse specialist and discuss how she can help you.' [Supportive and Prescriptive]

Mrs Black: 'Oh I don't want to make a fuss.'

Adam: 'You are not making a fuss. This is her area of expertise. I will contact her and arrange an appointment for you. I will also inform your husband's doctor, he may review his medication.' [Prescriptive]

Mrs Black: 'Thank you Adam.'

Adam: 'I also have information regarding the local carers' group. Are you aware of this group?' [Informative and Catalytic]

Mrs Black: 'No I don't know about it – what does it do?'

Adam: It is a support group, usually about eight to ten people who, like you, care for their partners or parents. It takes place every Tuesday at 2pm for an hour. They have a very good reputation. I have some leaflets about the group for you to read. If you have any questions, please let me know.' [Informative]

Overlapping of categories

All six categories are independent of one another and have a specific intention or purpose; there are also significant areas of overlap between the categories, for example informative interventions that are confronting, prescriptive interventions that are catalytic, and others. When such overlap occurs, the intervention is then classified under the category, that covers its primary purpose, as illustrated in the following examples.

Informative intervention – confronting intervention

Nurse: 'Your community mental health nurse told me that you did not attend the day centre.'

On its own, this intervention could be considered as an informative intervention whereby the mental health nurse is informing the client about what she/he knows. However, looking at the intervention within the following context, the intervention is identified according to its primary purpose or intention, which in this instance is to challenge the client in a supportive way; therefore, the same verbal intervention is a confronting intervention.

It is important to remember that the nurse's body language will also be an influencing factor.

Client: 'I don't like going to the day centre, there's nothing to do, and it's boring.'

Nurse: 'Your community mental health nurse told me that you did not attend the day centre.'

Client: 'Well I went to a day centre years ago.'

Prescriptive intervention – catalytic intervention

Nurse: 'Describe what it was like for you when you felt the urge to cut yourself.'

As it is, this intervention illustrates that the mental health nurse is directing the client to describe her recent experience of self-harm. Therefore, this intervention could be described as a prescriptive intervention; however, on examining the intervention within the following context and its primary purpose, which is to encourage the client to explore her experience of self-harm in greater depth, the verbal intervention is a catalytic intervention.

Client: 'I tried to stop myself, but I couldn't. I got the blades from my father's razor.'

Nurse: 'That must have been really difficult for you.'

Client: 'It was . . . it was very difficult. I feel really bad now.'

Nurse: 'Describe what it was like for you when you feel the urge to cut yourself.'

Client: 'I feel numb inside, I need to cut myself to feel alive.'

Degenerate use of interventions

An intervention is described as 'degenerate' not in the sense of being malicious, but more that it is misguided due to a lack of awareness, or lack of experience or training (Heron, 2001). As a result, the intervention may not be appropriate and/or effective. There are four kinds of degenerate intervention:

- unsolicited interventions
- manipulative interventions
- compulsive interventions
- unskilled interventions.

Unsolicited interventions

Unsolicited interventions are interventions whereby the practitioner intervenes before checking whether the client wishes to enter into the interaction with the practitioner. In such instances, the practitioner undermines the client's personal autonomy and responsibility. For example, the client is informed at the MDT meeting that he is to be discharged in two days. The mental health nurse approaches him and says, 'You might want to inform your family that you are going home tomorrow.' A more appropriate response might be to preface the intervention with the following:

'I heard that you are going home tomorrow, may I suggest something to you?' Pause to offer the client the opportunity to accept or reject the intervention.
Client: 'Yes, what is it?'
Nurse: 'You might want to inform your family that you are going home tomorrow.'

Manipulative interventions

These are interventions whereby the interventions are motivated by the practitioner's self-interest regardless of the interest of the client. In their worst form, such interventions are quite conscious and, deliberate, and are ways of using other people for their own self-interest. In practice, however, manipulative interventions may be motivated by practitioners' self-interest more often than we would like to admit, for example Jane, the mental health nurse, is about to finish her shift. She is tired and is looking forward to her weekend off. A client approaches her and says 'I feel very anxious, can I talk to you?' Jane reluctantly agrees to talk to the client. Although she listens to the client, she does not probe or ask any questions to gain a better understanding of the client's anxiety; instead she advises the client to 'Lie on your bed and practise your breathing exercises, you will feel much better.' It is 5pm, Jane leaves the ward on time.

Compulsive interventions

As the name suggests, these are interventions whereby the practitioner uses specific interventions compulsively. The compulsive helper may be unaware of their desire or need to help others, and as a result they make too many decisions for people about what they should do, how they do it and when they do it, while ignoring the person's autonomy and responsibility to choose what she or he wants to do. The compulsive helper usually has a limited range of interventions, which are frequently misused in practice. For example, the mental health nurse who compulsively prescribes or tells the client what she/he should do:

* 'You should say this . . .'
* 'You need to do more exercise'
* 'You should take your medication'
* 'You need to lose weight'

Unskilled interventions

Unskilled interventions occur when the practitioner is incompetent, or is not trained to carry out a specific intervention(s). For example, it is highly unlikely that a novice nurse will be competent to use cathartic interventions when working with a client who has had a recent bereavement. Equally, a qualified nurse who has much experience in adult mental health may be incompetent and untrained to use specific interventions in a different and new area of mental health practice, for example CAMS (Child and Adolescent Mental Health Services).

Learning to use the six categories

Learning how to use the Six Category framework, and use it effectively, will present different learning opportunities and challenges for the mental health nurse. Given the uniqueness of each client–nurse relationship, each interaction will require different communication skills and interventions, based on the purpose of the interaction, the context of the therapeutic encounter and the nurse's level of competence. Learning to use the Six Category framework does not mean the mental health nurse is learning a particular method of counselling (Heron, 2001). Instead, he/she is acquiring a set of therapeutic interventions to develop and shape into his/her style and repertoire of interpersonal skills as a mental health nurse. Having the opportunity to use the different categories in clinical practice can increase mental health nurses' confidence and efficacy. For some nurses, some of the interventions, particularly those within the authoritative group, may be familiar and therefore easier to use, whereas other interventions, for example catalytic and cathartic, may be new and, as with all new learning, will require time and ongoing practice. Learning how to use these skills can best be achieved by observing your mentor or other ward staff along with practising with friends or colleagues. For the mental health nurse, the challenge is to:

- be equally proficient in a wide range of interventions in each of the categories
- know what category s/he is using and why at any given time
- be able to move skilfully from one type of intervention to any other as the developing situation and purpose of the interaction requires
- know when to lead and when to follow the client, in other words whether to be authoritative or facilitative.

Clinical scenario

The following scenarios illustrate an interaction whereby the mental health nurse moves from one category to another, as and when the situation and purpose of the interaction requires.

Example I – Interaction between nurse and client

Zoe, a second-year nurse was sitting in the day room playing Scrabble with Sarah. Sarah is 21 years old and was admitted to the ward following an overdose. Both Zoe and Sarah enjoy playing Scrabble and competing with each other. It also provides an opportunity for Sarah to talk about various issues that were causing her concern, in particular her recent weight gain due to her current medication.

Sarah: 'I hate taking these tablets.'

Zoe: 'What do you hate about the tablets?' [Catalytic]

Sarah: 'They make you fat, I don't want to put on weight.'

Zoe: 'How much weight have you put on?' [Catalytic]

Sarah: 'I don't know, I haven't weighed myself, but my clothes are getting tight. I keep eating, I can't stop.'

Zoe: 'That must be so annoying for you. I know I hate having to watch my weight, it's difficult.' [Supportive]

Sarah: 'Yes it is.' [Starts to cry] 'I am sorry.'

Zoe: 'It's OK to cry.' [Cathartic] 'One of the side effects of your antidepressants is an increased appetite.' [Informative] 'I will weigh you and that will give us a baseline. I will get the dietician to see you tomorrow to discuss your diet. Your doctor will be here later this morning; I will tell him and ask him to talk to you about it.' [Prescriptive]

Sarah: 'Thanks Zoe.'

Example 2 – Interaction between nurse and family member

At the day hospital, Lydia asks to speak to Harry, a third-year nurse, about her son Toby who is 22 and attends the day hospital twice a week. She is worried that he is not taking his medication as he has been verbally aggressive over the weekend. Harry invites Lydia to a quiet and private area of the day hospital, free from distractions, to listen to the person.

Harry: 'Hi Lydia, how are you?'

Lydia: 'Thanks for talking to me; I know you are short of staff and very busy.'

Harry: What's the matter, you look worried?' [Catalytic]

Lydia: 'It's Toby; he stayed with me at the weekend.'

Harry: 'How did that go?' [Catalytic]

Lydia: 'He got angry. I don't think he is taking his medication. He kept shouting at me.'

Harry: 'OK, I am sorry to hear that.' [Supportive] 'Tell me what happened from the time he arrived at your house.' [Prescriptive]

Lydia: 'He was supposed to arrive at 6pm. He came two hours late so his dinner was ruined. I was really upset as I wanted us to eat together. He said he was with his mates.'

Harry: 'So you were disappointed and upset.' [Supportive] 'What happened when he arrived?' [Catalytic]

Lydia: 'Oh I lost it. I started shouting at him, I said things I probably shouldn't have but he's always messing me about.'

Harry: 'What happened then?' [Catalytic]

Lydia: 'He stormed into his bedroom and swore at me.'

Harry: 'So it sounds as if the weekend started off with difficulty for both of you.' [Supportive]

Lydia: 'Yea, I suppose I didn't make it easy, shouting at him. I know it's hard for him. He is afraid his mates will drop him because he has mental health problems and was in as he calls it "a lunny bin".'

(continued)

Harry: 'It's difficult for him; unfortunately there is still a lot of stigma about mental health problems/illness.' [Informative]

Lydia: 'Yes, I know. I haven't told my immediate family or my best friend about Toby's admission to hospital.'

Harry: 'Because?' [Catalytic]

Lydia: 'I am sure they would be supportive, but I am afraid they will look at Toby differently. I know it sounds crazy, but I am also afraid they will think it's my fault.'

Harry: 'It must be difficult for you, not being able to share your concerns with people who might be able to support you.' [Supportive]

Practice exercise: analysis of an interaction

The aim of this activity is to help you to monitor, select and review your use of Heron's six categories in clinical practice.

Think of a recent interaction that took place during your clinical placement.

- When you have chosen your interaction, reflect on and answer the following questions.
- You may wish to write brief notes about your thoughts, feelings, observations, questions in your reflective journal and use them to discuss with your mentor.
- It is important to note that some of the questions may not apply to your interaction, and, in such instances, we suggest that you adapt the question(s) accordingly.
- We are aware that the following questions are by no means exhaustive and you may wish to add further questions.

Question	Answer
What was my primary intention of this interaction?	
What intervention(s) did I use during this interaction?	
Which intervention(s) were useful?	
Which intervention(s) were less useful?	
What intervention(s) did I use too much?	
What intervention(s) did I use too little and for what reasons?	
What other intervention(s) could I have used?	
What did I like about my intervention?	
What did I not like about my intervention(s)?	
What factors influenced my intervention(s) and how?	
What have I learnt from this interaction?	
What intervention(s) do I need to develop?	

Conclusion

This chapter has outlined the principles and practice of Heron's Six Category helping framework. We believe that this communication framework provides a flexible and user-friendly tool for all mental health nurses, and in particular the novice mental health nurse, to develop their ongoing knowledge and interpersonal skills, which can be used in various clinical encounters. As with all skills-based learning, it is not enough to learn simply the specific interventions; they must be applied in practice where real learning takes place. In addition, learning how to use the six categories effectively and with confidence requires time, ongoing practice and, more importantly, a willingness to be open to inquiry and feedback about your therapeutic effectiveness in practice.

Reflective questions

1 Which of the authoritative categories do you find the most challenging and why?
2 Which of the facilitative categories do you find the most challenging and why?
3 Drawing on your clinical experience, which categories have you observed being used most in clinical practice? Give examples for each category.
4 Which two categories would you like to become more skilled in using within the next three months, and for what reasons?

6 Communicating across cultures

Britain is invariably described as one of the most ethnically diverse societies in the Western world. In the course of caring for members of society, nurses will come into contact with black and minority ethnic (BME) people with diverse cultures, beliefs and languages from around the world. Mental health nurses have an important role in delivering equality in mental health services through appropriate and effective culturally capable practice. This chapter will examine the concept of culture and its role in relation to mental health nursing. We will also outline various approaches to build on nurses' ability to become more culturally competent in communicating with a diverse multi-ethnic population.

Learning outcomes

By the end of this chapter, you should be better able to:

1 Describe the concept of culture
2 Demonstrate an understanding of the role of culture in relation to mental health nursing
3 Examine some of the issues and challenges for nurses when working with interpreters in mental health
4 Demonstrate communicating across cultures in clinical practice

Understanding culture

Culture is a difficult concept to define. This is further compounded by the numerous definitions throughout the literature, which are often used in different contexts as though there were a shared understanding of the terminology used. It is important therefore to be explicit about what is meant by the term culture, and more importantly, its importance to mental health nursing. In 1978, Madeline Leininger, an American nurse anthropologist, wrote a key text on the theory and practices of transcultural nursing (Leininger, 1978). In this book, Leininger stressed the importance of including culture as a fundamental component of patient-centred nursing care and nursing curricula, which she defined as 'the learned and transmitted knowledge about a particular culture with its values, beliefs, rules of behavior, and life-style practices that guides a designated group in their thinking and actions in patterned ways'

(Leininger, 1978, p.491). This definition suggests that culture is learned and is neither inherited nor static. A more recent definition describes culture as a shared set of learned behaviours, values, beliefs, norms, assumptions, perceptions, customs, social interactions and the world-view of a particular group (Allot, 2005). Culture is universal in that humans cannot exist apart from culture (Agar, 1994). In any given society, culture may therefore be regarded as the blueprint that defines the roles, relationships, rights and obligations of its members. The following example illustrates how the nurse became more aware of a client's cultural background and its impact on the client's wellbeing.

Clinical scenario

An English woman, Mrs Cohen, was admitted to the ward following the recent death of her older sister. On admission, she was withdrawn, uncommunicative, low in mood and refused to eat. Over time, Mrs Cohen's mood and wellbeing improved and she became much more communicative. Niamh, a newly qualified nurse, had built a good therapeutic relationship with Mrs Cohen. Niamh was aware that Mrs Cohen was Jewish and had ordered Kosher meals as requested. One day while watching TV, Mrs Cohen became extremely distressed, shouting 'turn it off; turn it off, all my family died there'. Later, Niamh gently asked if she wished to talk about the incident. Mrs Cohen explained slowly and with great difficulty that she and her sister, Ruth, came to the UK during WWII. Although she was very young, she remembered saying goodbye to her parents as they boarded the ship in Poland. A few years later, a close family friend told her and Ruth that their parents and other family members had died in a concentration camp. She remembered crying and being comforted by Ruth, who said 'I will look after you.' She described how her sister had always looked out for her. Mrs Cohen apologized for shouting and said, 'I know the Holocaust was many years ago but I can't forget it, it's part of me.' Niamh thanked Mrs Cohen for sharing her experiences with her. Throughout the day, Niamh thought about the interaction. She reflected on her own culture, in particular her religion and what it meant to her both as a person and as a nurse. She also thought about her nursing interventions and whether she paid sufficient attention to clients' cultural background and their specific needs beyond their dietary or spiritual needs.

Within the literature, various writers often use the terms 'multicultural', 'multiracial' and 'multiethnic' as though they are interchangeable. Multiculturalism argues for the promotion of tolerance and understanding between different cultural groups and traditions (Papadopoulous, 2001). Some writers in this field have criticized the term multicultural because it avoids addressing the role of racism in social and health inequality (Culley, 2001). The term 'race' is often associated with biology and refers to differences in the genetic composition of members of a particular race, sharing features such as skin colour (Giger and Davidhizar, 1999). In contrast, the term 'ethnicity' is socially constructed and generally refers to the cultural practices and attitudes that characterize a given group of people. Characteristics such as language, religion or social customs, which are often linked to a specific geographical territory, provide people in an ethnic group with a distinctive sense of identity (Culley and Dyson, 2001). Ethnic and racial groups often share biological and cultural similarities. The terms culture and ethnicity are often used interchangeably and, while there may be overlap, the concepts are not synonymous. Within ethnic groups, factors such as gender, age, education, religion and socio-economic status result in cultural diversity within an ethnic group. Furthermore, sometimes the term 'ethnic' is often used to refer to ethnic minority groups; however 'everybody is ethnic and belongs to a group' (Byrne 2008, p.387). To sum up, culture:

- is learned
- is shared
- is constantly changing
- transmits meaning
- defines
  - values
  - world-view
  - norms of behaviour
  - roles and relationships
  - beliefs and behaviour or practices
  - rights and obligations.

Practice exercise

Using the above characteristics of culture, identify how they apply to your own culture, giving specific examples where possible. Now, answer the following questions.

1 What have you learnt about your own culture from undertaking this exercise?
2 Have your cultural beliefs, practices and behaviours changed in the past ten years? If so, in what way?
3 What cultural beliefs, practices and behaviours are the same or different from those of your family of origin?

Culture and mental health

Issues of culture and health, and in particular mental health, are sensitive and the subject of much debate and controversy. The interplay between cultural factors and mental health has gained increasing attention and recognition over the years. Transcultural or cross-cultural psychiatry represents a shift from the traditional-generic psychiatry or Western model, which assumes that mental illness is universal irrespective of the person's ethnic background to an understanding of a multitude of cultural and social factors and their influence on mental health (Fernando, 2003). The mental health status and care of BME people are influenced by cultural factors originating from the ethnic minority group itself, mental health professionals, the mental health care system and society as a whole. However, there is widespread evidence that people from black and minority ethnic groups are reluctant to use health care services (Madhok et al., 1992) because they are dissatisfied with the quality of health care they receive, and believe it to be unequal, inequitable and insensitive to their needs (DH, 2005). Examples of unequal treatment of ethnic minorities abound in the literature. Generally, the main areas of disparity among different ethnic groups in mental health care concern the following:

- the mode of entry into psychiatric institutions
- the disease profile
- the treatment regimes.

As a result, BME people, compared to white people and larger ethnic groups (Bhui et al., 2003):

- are over-represented among inpatients
- have more complex pathways to specialist mental health care
- are more likely to experience compulsory and emergency admission to psychiatric services with police involvement.

Although there is evidence to support a strong association between ethnicity and mental health patterns, it is limited and offers few explanations for these observed relationships (Iley and Nazroo, 2001). Ethnicity in itself never determines the person's health status. Further research is required to identify other causal factors, however some of the explanations for disparities among different ethnic groups in mental health include:

- racism
- cultural factors
- access to health services
- socio-economic factors
- genetic factors.

So far in this chapter we have outlined the concept of culture and its relationship with mental health. We will now look at the role culture and mental health nursing.

Culture and mental health nursing

The importance of a transcultural perspective to care has been recognized in nursing for several years. As previously stated, Leininger (1995) pioneered the development of transcultural or cross-cultural nursing in the USA. Transcultural nursing is built on the principle of cultural competence, which is defined as 'the process in which a healthcare provider continuously strives to achieve the ability to effectively work within the cultural context of a client' (Campinha-Bacote, 1999, p.203). Leininger's (1991) conceptual framework of transcultural nursing, known as the Sunrise Model, depicts the Theory of Culture Care Diversity and Universality. In mental health nursing, Campinha-Bacote (1999, 2003) developed a model of cultural competence to be used specifically for developing culturally responsive mental health care provision. This model comprises the components described below and is based on the premise that the development of the respective components helps the nurse to become more culturally competent and capable:

- cultural desire
- cultural awareness
- cultural knowledge
- cultural skills
- cultural encounter.

Model of cultural/diversity competence

Cultural desire	Refers to the nurse's: • motivation and commitment to engage in culturally competent care • willingness to accept difference and build on similarities • willingness to be open and willing to learn from others.
Cultural awareness	Refers to the nurse's: • awareness of the dynamics of culture and how culture shapes values and beliefs • awareness of his/her own values, beliefs, prejudices and practices in relation to diverse and minority groups • ability to examine his/her own cultural background in an effort to avoid the tendencies to ethnocentrism.
Cultural knowledge	Refers to the nurse: • continually acquiring information about diverse cultures • interacting with people of other cultures • gaining understanding and knowledge about clients' health-related values, meanings, beliefs, behaviour-patterns and their world-views • learning about physical, psychological, psychiatric and social variations among peoples.
Cultural skills	Refers to the nurse: • collecting relevant cultural information in a culturally sensitive manner • determining the client's nursing care needs within his/her cultural context • drawing up an individual care plan that addresses the client's perspective • implementing nursing interventions based on the client's cultural assessment.
Cultural encounters	Refers to the nurse: • Working with the client's family/carer/community.

Source: Based on Campinha-Bacote (1999)

Cultural awareness is the first step towards cultural competence. Becoming aware of one's own values, beliefs, prejudices and practices in relation to BME people is essential, albeit at times uncomfortable and challenging, in order to identify, confront and eliminate one's biases, stereotypes and prejudices. It helps the nurse to undertake the journey from ethnocentrism (the perception that one's own culture is best) to ethno-relativity – the appreciation of the equal value of all cultures (Byrne, 2008). However, the lack of attention to the role played by the nurse's own ethnicity and cultural perspective in nursing interventions, including communication skills, which seem to demonstrate an inherent ethnocentricity, has been criticized (Price and Cortis, 2000).

Nurses' experiences of caring for BME service users have been evaluated in a variety of settings (Narayanasamy, 2003). While nurses acknowledged that clients have cultural needs, particularly in relation to language, religion, diet and family visitors, these needs were generally not well addressed. Transcultural nursing and cultural competence has been recognized and its implementation has received much attention, especially in the area of nursing education (Canales and Bowers, 2001). However, there is a lack of empirical evidence to support claims that culturally competent nursing care facilitates the development of positive health outcomes for ethnic minorities and helps reduce ethnic health disparities (Warren, 2003). Notwithstanding this, we believe that culturally competent nursing care is paramount for effective communication with clients from diverse cultural backgrounds.

Communicating across cultures

Communication and the development of the nurse–client helping relationship are central to cross-cultural mental health nursing. Culture comprises every verbal or behavioural system that transmits meaning. Language and cultural differences can make it difficult for the nurse and client to achieve effective and therefore therapeutic communication, as well as a positive helping relationship. This may be because the nurse does not understand the client's language or feel skilled when communicating with clients from BME groups. Knowledge of the different rules and styles of communicating among BME clients is essential. This is addressed in Chapter 2, which we recommend you revisit while reading this chapter. We also suggest that you take a look at Chapter 7, which focuses on the key components of engaging in a helping relationship. We believe that the same principles apply to developing helping relationships with people from BME groups. The next section addresses communication via the use of a third person, an interpreter.

Working with interpreters

In today's society, there is increasing need for mental health nurses to work with interpreters. Many service users of mental health are primary speakers of languages other than English. Issues of good cross-cultural communication are therefore becoming increasingly important within health services, and language is a central facet of this (Bischoff et al., 2003). However, despite its importance, coverage of this subject has received little attention in the literature in general and in mental health nursing in particular. Without a common language, people are unable to communicate their requirements to mental health nurses, with negative consequences for their mental health and wellbeing, treatment and outcomes (Tribe and Morrissey, 2003). For the client, this may also result in problems of access to mental health services and their different cultural needs not being met. Furthermore, the services offered might not be appropriate, culturally sensitive or meaningful to the client. The inability to speak the dominant or host language is likely to exacerbate the client's feelings of exclusion and mental distress. Communication in this situation between mental health nurses and the client cannot take place without an interpreter. Working with interpreters in mental health helps nurses to develop better ways of helping clients who need an interpreter.

The value and role of interpreters

When the client and nurse do not speak the same language, a potentially challenging communication barrier must be overcome. An interpreter often provides an important link between the two parties and their contribution should be respected accordingly. The benefits of using interpreters for non-English-speaking clients are well documented. Several studies have noted that when the client and nurses can speak the same language or have access to qualified interpreters, there is improved client satisfaction, quality of communication and compliance with health regimes (Eyton et al., 2002; Lee et al., 2002).

Interpreters offer a valuable and skilful service, and can play an important and indispensable role by:

- bridging the gap between the client and mental health nurse
- ensuring that non-English-speaking clients are not restricted from accessing health services, including mental health and social services provision
- enabling mental health assessments to be carried out.

Models of interpreting

In mental health, 'the task of the interpreter is a complex and sophisticated one requiring a range of skills beyond just the ability to speak two languages fluently' (Tribe and Morrissey, 2003, p.208). Translating between languages can in effect mean translating between two separate world-views. Language is multi-faceted, dynamic and constantly changing to incorporate new words or societal changes. Languages are not interchangeable. Words in one language might not exist in another and may reflect a culture or societal context, or indeed may get lost in the translation (Hoffman, 1998). Time frames and the patterns and placing of tenses do not correspond across some languages (Tribe,

2004). Various languages do not always distinguish between present, perfect and pluperfect tenses, and grammatical constructions can differ in a number of ways. The following example illustrates how words to describe mood states might not exist in another language.

Words to describe emotions

The English language has a large range of words to describe mood states, for example a person who is feeling depressed might use one or more of the following: upset; gloomy; melancholy; despondent; miserable; morbid; dispirited; sad; unhappy; low; down and many more.

So imagine the following description of this person's mood following the recent break-up of a relationship, 'I feel down since I broke up with my boyfriend, but I am not going to let it make me miserable. As far as I can remember, I have always felt a bit low, but I never get depressed, I am just sad now that it didn't work out'.

Similarly, a person who is feeling angry might use the following words to describe their anger: 'I am so pissed off, my parents never visit me. I am fed up with them telling me what to do. They don't understand what it's like having to take these tablets. The tablets make you feel irritable and angry all the time. The more I think of it, the crosser I get. Actually, I am furious with them for not understanding.'

In many non-European languages, no such vocabulary exists to describe different moods. It is important to be mindful of this when working with interpreters and to clarify the meaning of words, particularly when such descriptions are used as diagnostic features, for example depression in Western society (Rack, 1982).

There are four basic models of interpreting, which are described below. Each one of these approaches will be used in particular circumstances.

1 **The linguistic mode** (Cushing, 2003):
   - the interpreter tries to interpret as far as is possible word-for-word, and adopts a neutral and distanced position
   - is best suited when factual information is required and any psychological or emotional meaning is not seen as largely relevant, for example in a medico-legal setting.
2 **The psychotherapeutic or constructionist mode** (Raval, 2003):
   - the interpreter is primarily concerned with the meaning/feeling of the words to be conveyed rather than word-for-word interpretation
   - is most useful when working within a psychotherapeutic context where the meaning/feeling of emotions and words is essential
   - is best used if there is to be a series of meetings rather than a one-off assessment

- allows the interpreter more flexibility to ensure that the client's meaning is accurately conveyed
- requires a higher level of responsibility, training and trust between the client, mental health nurse and the interpreter.

3 **The advocate or community interpreter** (Razban, 2003):
- takes on the role of advocate for the client either at the individual or community level, and represents the client's interests beyond interpreting language
- ensures that the specific health or cultural views and needs of a community or faith group are understood and met, for example Sudanese Muslim women
- assists clients to negotiate or challenge the health care offered at the individual level and service provision level
- is employed in Britain throughout many parts of the National Health Service to try to ensure that there is some equity of health provision and appropriate service provision regardless of clients' language skills.

4 **Cultural broker/bicultural worker** (Tribe, 1998):
- is concerned with interpreting cultural and contextual variables as well as the words
- this model is based on the view that to understand the client's emotional world it is important to understand their context and cultural worldview
- best used when working in the domain of psychological and mental health
- requires trust, open communication and shared responsibility between the client, interpreter and mental health nurse
- most useful when the interpreter is experienced, and the mental health nurse has developed experience and expertise with working with interpreters and feels comfortable working in a more collaborative manner.

Working with interpreters in mental health: good practice principles

Working with an interpreter in mental health changes the helping relationship: what is traditionally a dyadic relationship becomes a triadic one. Communicating through a third person is a challenging task for all involved in this non-traditional triad; however, it can also improve the practice of mental health nursing and hopefully the delivery of care. If the best outcomes of the work are to be maximized, these challenges need to be considered before undertaking clinical work using interpreters (Tribe, 1998). The following principles are not intended to be a definitive or exhaustive list but instead are aimed at helping you work more effectively with interpreters in your area of practice (Tribe and Morrissey, 2004). We recognize that the provision and availability of trained and qualified interpreters, and their contractual agreements, will vary in different mental health settings throughout the UK.

Working with interpreters in mental health: good practice principles

Accessing an interpreter	Familiarize yourself with the interpreters' service in your area of practice, their model of interpreting and policies, particularly in relation to confidentiality.
Choosing an interpreter	Use interpreters who are trained and experienced in working in mental health, when possible.
	Find out the client's first language and try to request an interpreter who speaks this language, ideally from the same country, and when necessary the same dialect.
	Do not assume that someone who speaks a language can speak and understand all its dialects.
	This is particularly significant in a mental health context, where the client's exact meaning and intent will be extremely important.
	Try to match an interpreter and client for gender, age and religion, particularly if this is relevant to the meeting, for example where it concerns a sexual assault or domestic violence.
	Try to use the same interpreter throughout, especially if you are planning to see the client a number of times. This will facilitate the process for all the participants.
Allocating time	Allow plenty of time for meeting/consultation with the interpreter, which can take longer, as twice as many words have to be spoken.
Preparing for translation	Establish a good working agreement with the interpreter at the outset. Discuss how you will work together and the following issues: model of translation, confidentiality, purpose of interview and any other factors that are relevant to the interview.
The bilingual meeting	Seating arrangements: some recommend a triangle arrangement, with the interpreter closer to the client.
	Use direct, short sentences.
	Avoid using technical or specialist terminology whenever possible. If this is unavoidable, try to ensure that the interpreter is familiar with the terminology, to minimize the potential for misunderstandings.
	Avoid using colloquialisms, slang or metaphors, as these tend to be culturally embedded, for example 'Are you feeling a bit under the weather?' 'It's six of one and half a dozen of the other.'
	Pace what you say. The interpreter has to remember what has been said, translate it, and then convey it to the other person. If you speak for too long, the interpreter may struggle to remember the first part of what you said.

(continued)

	Look at the client when you speak.
Debriefing	Spend a few minutes with the interpreter after each session reviewing how you worked together, and discuss any other pertinent aspects.
	Check that the interpreter is OK after the interview, particularly if the nature of the conversation was emotionally challenging, for example sexual abuse, suicidal behaviour. Offer available support if needed.
	Invite interpreter to give his or her impression of the meeting and your work together. Clarify any relevant cultural issues arising from the session.
Respecting and protecting client	Finally, but most importantly...
	Avoid using family members. They do not make good interpreters as the accuracy of their translation may be compromised by their lack of objectivity, understanding, embarrassment or verbal ability.
	Best practice precludes the use of children to act as interpreters.

Source: Tribe and Morrissey (2004)

The following is an account of Paul's, a third-year student nurse, reflections on his experience of working with an interpreter, Mustapha, and a client, Ibrahim, who is from the Sudan.

Clinical scenario

Although it was my first time working with an interpreter, I had discussed and prepared for it with my mentor who has a lot of experience working with interpreters. I asked Mustapha if we could meet before the interview to discuss how we might undertake the interview. During this time, we discussed the purpose of the interview with the client, maintaining confidentiality and his model of interpretation. Mustapha explained that he sometimes translates literally, using a word-for-word translation, depending on what the client says. However, whenever there is not a similar word in English or Arabic, he would then give the overall meaning. Overall the interview went well although it was a strange experience speaking to the client through another person. I tried to look at the client when I spoke but I found this difficult. I am aware that at times I looked at Mustapha instead of Ibrahim. It was strange, when I asked a short question, for example 'How do you feel today?' Mustapha's translation into Arabic seemed to take a lot longer and he used a lot more words. At times, I felt excluded, particularly when Mustapha and Ibrahim were talking for what felt like a long time. I suspect this is how it must feel for Ibrahim, being surrounded by people who are unable to communicate in his language. I have never fully understood or appreciated how this must feel for the client, particularly if they are frightened and distressed.

Mustapha and I spent some time discussing our impression of the meeting and clarified any relevant cultural issues arising from the interview, for example the sense of shame associated with mental illness for the client and family. This was useful in understanding Ibrahim's family's reluctance to visit or engage with mental health services. Another valuable piece of learning for me concerned my preconceived beliefs about Mustapha's cultural background. I had assumed, incorrectly, that Mustapha was from the Sudan or another Arabic country. Instead, he told me that he was born and educated in France, his parents being British and Sudanese. I learnt never to assume! This experience has taught me about the importance of the interpreter's role and the need to work collaboratively.

Learning to be culturally competent and capable

The clinical setting provides a rich learning resource to become more culturally sensitive, competent and capable. However, exposure to BME clients alone is not the key to learning. Learning involves:

- acknowledging that our beliefs, values and reactions are programmed by our own culturally determined view of the world
- listening and attending to the client with a view to gathering a cultural understanding
- asking the client about his/her culture with a genuine interest and respect
- being culturally informed, consulting other sources of information – books, films, training, courses, etc.

However, as with all learning, it requires time, commitment and an open mindedness to examine one's own practice, thoughts, feelings and responses. This in turn puts pressure on nurses to engage in extra work. It is important that nurses do not set out to accumulate knowledge of all cultures, which given the huge number and variety of cultures in Britain is unrealistic. A more realistic perspective might be to get to know something of those specific cultures from which your clients most regularly come. Finally, it is important to be aware that what is written about cultural diversity reflects a description of broad cultural tendencies; the extent to which they are acceptable as truth and therefore applicable to the complete range of personalities has to be seriously questioned (Lago and Thompson, 1996). One culture does not fit all.

Practice exercise

The aim of this activity is for you to consider the broad cultural tendencies that people may have about your specific cultural/ethnic background. We would like you to reflect on the following questions and jot down your thoughts, ideas and feelings in your journal. Try to be as specific as possible in your answers, as illustrated below. You may also wish to spend some time reflecting on your answers with a colleague or your mentor.

Questions

1   What broad cultural tendencies do people have about your cultural/ethnic background in terms of language, religion, specific behaviours?
2   How do you feel hearing people say specific things about your culture?
3   How do you respond when people say specific things about your culture?
4   What aspects of your cultural/ethnic background would you like people to be more informed about?
5   What broad cultural tendencies do you have about the cultural/ethnic background of your clients in terms of language, religion, specific behaviours?

Conclusion

Communicating across cultures is essential in an ethnically diverse society. Mental health nurses have an important role in delivering equality in mental health services through appropriate and effective culturally capable practice. However, issues of culture in mental health are complex, sensitive and challenging. For the mental health nurse, being culturally sensitive and competent demands time, commitment and an openness to learn about one's own culture as well as that of others. Engaging in a process of learning about one's cultural self can help the mental health nurse to recognize, understand and predict his/her own behaviours, which hopefully will help nurses to gain insight and understanding of others' cultural positions through empathy.

Reflective questions

1   What cultural/ethnic beliefs/practices do you bring into your clinical work?
2   How might you respond if you thought one of your colleagues was practising in a racist manner?
3   What could you do to become more familiar with the different cultures of people from BME groups in your area of clinical practice?
4   What challenges might you face when working with interpreters in your area of clinical practice?

7 Professional helping relationships

Introduction

Mental health nursing consists of a professional helping relationship in which sound interpersonal skills are used to develop, sustain and end therapeutic encounters in a caring, competent and compassionate manner. In this chapter we will unpack the active ingredients of helping relationships by showing:

- the characteristics of professional helping relationships
- examining the attributes of effective and ineffective helpers
- how to create a helping relationship
- factors that affect the capacity of mental health nurses to achieve a helping relationship
- what are the activities involved in receiving help.

Learning outcomes

By the end of this chapter, you should be better able to:

- Describe the characteristics of person-centred care
- Describe how the core conditions of empathy, acceptance (unconditional positive regard) and genuineness may be demonstrated to create a helping relationship
- Identify the characteristics of a professional helping relationship
- Outline the attributes of effective helpers

Patient-centred care – what is it?

In mental health nursing, the concept of patient-centred care, also referred to as person-centred care, has gained increasing momentum during the last 20 years. Its value as a fundamental principle underpinning the planning and delivery of mental health care, and as an important component of the helping relationship, has been recognized and supported by the nursing profession and literature (NHS Modernisation Agency, 2003; Department of Health [DH], 2004). These initiatives were in response to the concerns raised about the quality of interactions between nurses and services users and their therapeutic value (Sainsbury Centre, 1998; Felton and Stickley, 2004). Patient-centred care as a concept is poorly understood in clinical practice. This is further compounded by the fact that the term patient-centred care is often used in different contexts as though there were an agreed and shared understanding of the terminology used. It is important therefore to be explicit about what is understood by the term patient-centred care and, more importantly, how it is translated into clinical practice.

Essentially, patient-centred care is a method of helping that is concerned with understanding the client or service user's needs, and engaging in a model of care based on shared decision making, so that the client can maintain and improve his/her wellbeing (Kitwood and Bredin, 1992). In mental health nursing, this involves putting people at the centre of nursing care (Barker, 2003). One example of a patient-centred theory based approach to nursing is the Tidal Model (Barker and Buchanan-Barker, 2005). As a model of care, it places much emphasis on developing a helping relationship based on respect, trust and collaboration with service users. However, the helping relationship between the nurse and the client does not just happen or should not be taken as a given. Instead, it is built with care over time and based on certain core values, which are essential, particularly if the nurse wants to develop a positive, supportive and therapeutic relationship with the client. While there is extensive literature on the concept of patient-centred care, much of it is theoretical. Few studies have examined how patient-centred care is applied in practice and, more significantly, its usefulness from clients' perspective. Nonetheless, studies concerning service user involvement in care, such as the Tidal Model, suggest that models of care based on a more participatory approach are increasing in practice (Cook et al., 2005) albeit slowly and in a piecemeal manner (Felton and Stickley, 2004).

Being person-centred

Person-centred therapy (PCT), originally known as client-centred therapy, was developed by the American psychologist, Carl Rogers, over half a century ago (Rogers 1961). Since then it has been adopted as a model of care in many health professions, including mental health nursing. Being person-centred is at the core of a professional helping relationship. In this case, the focus of mental health nursing is caring for the person who is on the receiving end of this care. Using a person-centred approach is based on the following principles and characteristics of a helping relationship.

A **person-centred nurse:**

- **Appreciates** that each person is uniquely influenced by their heredity, the environment in which they are raised, and the values, beliefs and behaviour influenced by the culture in which they were reared.
- **Believes** that most people strive to reach their optimal potential as much as possible in order to achieve their personal life goals. In this case the mental health nurse considers with the person what are their

life goals, and the part that the therapeutic encounter with the nurse will play in helping the person reach these goals.

- **Respects** the worth of people. In this instance, the mental health nurse seeks to demonstrate their commitment to the helping process by acknowledging that what is troubling the person is real to them. A good example of showing this is listening actively to the person by, for example, paying attention to what they are saying, making sure that what you are saying is matched by how you are behaving and taking care to clarify with the person what their experiences mean to them.
- **Behaves** genuinely. One of three main facets of being person-centred is genuineness (Rogers, 1961)–that is, the ability to show that your commitment to helping the person is real. You can do this by working collaboratively with them and not crowding them out of the therapeutic encounter, listening actively and taking time to allow them to present what is troubling them.
- **Enables** control to remain with the person. In this example, the mental health nurse acts a facilitator to help the person identify what is troubling them, possible solutions to overcome these troubles and evaluation of the impact of the solutions agreed with the person. Using the facilitative categories of Heron's (2001) six categories of intervention will be useful here. For example, one of Heron's facilitative categories is catalytic. In this, your role is enabling the person to retain control for change. You can show this through the use of statements such as: 'List the things that you think might help you overcome this problem.' See Chapter 5 for further examples of catalytic interventions.
- **Recognizes** people have basic needs and are motivated to meet these needs. Being mindful of Maslow's Hierarchy of Human Needs may help in this instance. Based on a seminal paper first published in 1943, Maslow believed that people had five main needs from the **basic needs** necessary for survival, for example food; **safety needs**, those that bring comfort, for example health; **psychological needs**, for example the need for love or to belong, sometimes referred to as love and belonging; **self-esteem**, that is respecting others, being respected by others and having self-confidence; **self-actualization**, the highest order of need, that is the ideal state the person is seeking for themselves (Maslow, 1970).
- **Realizes** that people's behaviour is communicating something about their feelings, beliefs, physical and mental state. This is an important part of being person-centred and is especially useful when you are confronted with behaviour you find challenging. For example, you can demonstrate this by using an approach called functional analysis. Functional analysis is an approach to assessment whereby you try to understand what the person's behaviour represents. You can show this by asking questions such as 'What do you think your behaviour is telling others about how you're feeling?' (Lindberg et al., 1983)

Practice exercise

Consider the seven examples of being a person-centred nurse. Now think of an example from your work with a person for whom you have been caring. Give an example of being person-centred:

- What was the situation exactly?
- What was the person's presenting problem(s)?
- What aspects of being person-centred did you use?
- What aspects of being person-centred did you not use, and for what reason?
- How did the person react?
- What aspects of being person-centred would you like to develop further and how might you achieve this?

The core conditions of a helping relationship

Rogers (1961) believed that if helpers created relationships with the three core conditions of genuineness, acceptance and empathy, then the people they were attempting to help would begin to understand aspects of themselves that were previously unknown to them. As a result, this would help clients to become more self-confident and autonomous, understand and accept others and be more able to cope adequately with their everyday living. Similarly, in mental health nursing, valuing the views and opinions of service users is considered essential to the therapeutic relationship (Anthony and Crawford, 2000). However, the context of care has the greatest potential to enhance or limit the person-centred care, highlighting that nurses not only have to balance different care approaches and values but often organizational values (Alexander and Bowers, 2004).

The three core conditions are essential regardless of the type of situation in which they are used, for example, whether they are used with a client in an acute admission ward or in the service user's home in the community. We will now describe the core conditions or skills as described by Carl Rogers of a helping relationship, paying particular attention to the skill of empathy, given its importance as an essential interpersonal skill in mental health nursing.

The core conditions are:

- empathy
- congruence
- unconditional positive regard.

Understanding empathy

Empathy, the ability to communicate an understanding of a client's world, is widely accepted as a crucial component for all helping relationships

(Reynolds and Scott, 2000). In mental health nursing, it is considered a fundamental communication skill for nurses and an essential ingredient for developing a therapeutic relationship with clients (Peplau, 1997). However, empathy is a difficult concept to define. At its simplest, it refers to 'the ability to perceive the world from another person's viewpoint and to take on that perspective while not losing one's own' (Stevenson, 2008, p.112). This involves experiencing the feelings of another without losing one's own identity, and responding accurately without being overwhelmed by these feelings. An empathetic helper will sense the feelings of the client but will not lose the 'as if' component, which protects the helper from being disabled by the pain or distress of the client. Furthermore, the helper can only sense what the client is feeling, even if he/she has experienced a similar situation, because the client's experience and feelings are unique to him/her. Using the metaphor of 'being in another person's shoes', which is often used to describe the concept of empathy, the nurse can only imagine what it is like or 'as if' he/she were in the other person's shoes; while at the same time being mindful not to get into the other person's shoes. The latter acts to protect the helper from being overwhelmed by the client's emotions or lose his/her ability to be objective and offer effective therapeutic help to the client. Being empathetic also requires the helper not only to be 'attuned' to the way the person is feeling but also to convey that understanding to the client. As an interpersonal skill, empathy therefore involves the nurse's ability to undertake the following.

- Listen to gain a deeper understanding *with* the person as opposed to *about* the person. For example, listening with interest to the client and at the client's pace, rather than listening with interest to satisfy one's own self-interest.
- Understand the person's outer and inner worlds from their frame of reference as opposed to the nurse's frame of reference. For example, understanding what is happening for the client in relation to his external world, such as his/her social network, family or work, as well as what the client is feeling or experiencing internally at that time. This is what is often referred to in the literature as staying within 'the client's frame of reference'. In contrast, the nurse's frame of reference refers to what the nurse thinks or believes.
- Enter into the life of another and accurately perceive feeling and meaning.
- Live temporary in the client's life, without making judgements.
- Communicate your sense of the client's world back to the client – that is, using verbal and non-verbal skills to convey your sense of what you have heard back to the client, as illustrated in the following example: 'It looks like you're feeling very upset today. It seems as if you were very hurt by your father's response to your overdose.'

The above components of using the skill of empathy highlight the complexity of the empathetic process, which adds to the confusion about the meaning of empathy. Empathy is a multidimensional and multiphase construct, and has variously been conceptualized as a behaviour, personality dimension and an experienced emotion, as described below (Mac Kay et al., 1990):

- a behaviour, for example interpersonal skills such as listening, communicating back your sense of the client's world, non-verbal communication
- a personality dimension, for example an attitude or human quality or trait
- an experienced emotion, for example feeling what you sense the client is feeling.

We will now look briefly at some models of empathy, which tend to focus on the different stages of the empathetic process or the components of empathy.

Models of empathy

As a stage model, Barret-Lennard's (1981) multidimensional cyclical model of empathy comprises three phases, which consist of the following.

Cyclical model of empathy

- Phase 1: The helper is engaged in the inner process of empathetic listening to the client who is expressing him/herself, reasoning and understanding
- Phase 2: The helper tries to convey empathetic understanding of the client's experiences
- Phase 3: The client's response and awareness of the helper's communication

Source: Barret-Lennard (1981)

As the interaction continues, phase 1, which is the core feature, is repeated, followed by phases 2 and 3. The interactive sequence of the different phases leads to further expression by the client and is facilitated by the helper's empathetic listening and ability to convey empathetic understanding of the client's experience through communication. As a result, the client learns to change when the helper is able to communicate genuineness and understanding of the client's current feelings (Rogers, 1990). The helper's ability to convey an understanding through his/her communication to the client suggests that empathy is a skill and ability rather than an innate quality possessed by some person (Morse et al., 1994; Reynolds and Scott, 1999). This suggests that, similar to other communication skills, the skill of empathy can be learnt.

Morse et al. (1992) focused on the components of empathy rather than the stages of empathy, and identified four components of empathy – moral, emotive, cognitive and behavioural – which are described as follows:

Components of empathy

Component	Description of component
Emotive	The helper's ability to subjectively experience and share in another person's internal feelings
Moral	An internal altruistic force that motivates the practice of empathy
Cognitive	The helper's cognitive ability to identify and understand another person's feelings and perspective from an objective stance
Behavioural	The helper's communicative response to convey understanding of the other person's perspective

Source: Morse et al. (1992)

Although empathy contains many components, it is difficult to determine whether these components are interrelated, and/or the extent to which each component contributes more or less to behaviours that foster the development of an effective therapeutic helping relationship in mental health practice. Having examined what is meant by the skill of empathy, we will now examine the skill of sympathy, which is often misconstrued as empathy in clinical practice.

Empathy or sympathy?

Sympathetic responses are often described as empathy. Empathy, however, is not sympathy. In contrast, sympathy is used in everyday communication. A sympathetic response is a verbal and non-verbal expression of concern, reassurance or expression of consolation shown by the helper with regard to the person's problem or situation (Morse et al., 1992). It may be defined as the helper's expression of feeling '*for*' the person as opposed to '*with*' the person. As a communication skill, sympathy, which is a first-level empathetic response, conveys the helper's understanding and recognition of the client's situation. First-level or basic empathetic responses are recognized as important for developing rapport and trust in all helping relationships (Freshwater, 2003), as illustrated by the following examples:

- 'I am sorry to hear that you have been feeling so depressed'
- 'I am sorry that things didn't work out for you in the hostel'
- 'I am sorry to hear of your mum's death'
- 'You have had such a difficult time caring for your husband'
- 'You have had a lot to deal with this year'

When nurses are sympathetic, clients perceive that their experiences and/or feelings are being acknowledged and validated. However, communication responses such as sympathy, pity and commiseration have been devalued and viewed as non-therapeutic in the nursing literature. Expressing sympathy however, has a place in helping relationships; it 'can make clients feel understood, comforted and cared for as a person because the nurse has recognised how they may be feeling' (Morse et al., 1992, p.812). However, similar to using other communication skills, when using a sympathetic response, it is important to be aware of one's body language, the tone of the response, timing and context that can affect the therapeutic effectiveness of the intervention. While sympathetic responses offer therapeutic value, albeit limited, mental health nurses need to develop and acquire greater emotional and empathetic responses in order to provide more effective and therapeutic outcomes with their clients.

The use of empathy in practice

Throughout the extensive literature on empathy and therapeutic relationships, there is a widely held view that empathy is a fundamental component of all helping relationships, including medicine, psychology and nursing. In mental health nursing, several theorists have advocated the use of empathy as a potent and powerful interpersonal skill, which contributes to the achievement of positive outcomes for clients (Peplau, 1997; Barker, 2003; Freshwater, 2003). While there is considerable research to support such claims, evidence concerning the efficacy of empathy in the interpersonal process is inconclusive. Nevertheless, substantial cumulative evidence supports the relationship between empathy and the ability to help another person (Mac Kay et al., 1990; Fleuren et al., 1998). However, despite its prominence and relevance to clinical nursing, the ability to offer empathy is lacking among many helping professionals, including mental health nurses (Squier, 1990; Williams, 1992). Sadly, the low level of empathy reported indicates that many professionals are simply not as helpful as they ought to be (Reynolds and Scott, 2000). Without empathy, the nurse's ability to help the client will be reduced. In mental health nursing, the absence or lack of empathy is likely to interfere with the efficacy of the helping relationship and as a result have potential negative consequences for clients. Mental health nursing is about helping people; in order to fulfil this aim; nurses need not only to be able to demonstrate empathy but also at a level at which they can carry out the following interventions:

- access accurately the needs and problems of clients from a client-centred perspective
- demonstrate empathetic understanding of the client's concern.

If nurses fail to demonstrate empathy with their clients, the outcome of the helping relationship will be hindered and have potential negative consequences for clients. More specifically, it is unlikely that the following will take place for both members of the helping dyad:

- nurses will be able to understand clients' experiences and needs, as experienced by them and as a result help them to cope effectively

- nurses will be able provide clients with what they need, which is likely to contribute to delayed recovery
- clients will be able to trust nurses in an open two-way relationship, if they do not perceive that their situation or experience is understood
- clients who need to be understood will be understood, or may feel understood.

Several reasons have been put forward to explain the low level of empathy among helping professionals, including mental health nurses. Understanding these factors is particularly significant for nurse educators and clinicians, particularly given the widely accepted view that empathy is an essential requisite to effective therapeutic relationships and is essential at the outset of all helping relationships (Mac Kay et al., 1990). While there is limited research that describes factors that prevent or limit nurses' ability to use empathy, the following factors have been identified, which militate against the use of empathy in clinical practice (Williams, 1992; Reynolds and Scott, 2000). Overall, these factors consist of nurses' skills, nurse education and the culture of the organizational setting.

- Staffing levels, for example there may be limited time for nurses to listen to clients.
- Nurses' educational experience, for example nurses may lack the necessary communication skills and confidence to use empathy, such as empathetic listening, as well as the capacity to discuss and contain clients' feelings, or help them to focus on areas of concern, as perceived by clients.
- Professional socialization, for example nurses' tendency to focus on nurse-centred practices rather than patient-centred care, and focus on diagnosis and symptoms rather than clients' narratives and experiences.
- Organizational system or culture, for example if the practice of the clinical setting is more about getting the work done, which can contribute to the busy nurse syndrome, then it is unlikely that a patient-centred model of care will be adopted, and empathetic responses will occur.

Clinical scenario

The following is an account of the reflections of Rachel, a third-year nurse, who subsequently recognized that she unwittingly manipulated her interactions with a client to avoid discussing the client's feelings. Rachel had developed a good relationship with John. Over time, he had begun to trust her and slowly talk about his fears and concerns for the future. John was 56 years old and spent many years of his adult life as an inpatient in various mental health hospitals. As a result, he had lost contact with his children, whom he missed very much. One day, John showed Rachel an old photo of himself and his two sons. As he looked at the photo, his eyes filled with tears. Although Rachel felt privileged that John had shared this memory with her, she felt a deep sense

(continued)

of sadness for John and was afraid that she might begin to cry in front of him. She also felt a sense of helplessness; she did not know what to say or do *'to fix it'*. She recalled a sense of panic at the time and quickly thanked John for showing her the photo. She then asked him if he wanted to watch football on the TV. He put his photo away and said he would in a while. Rachel said 'I know you enjoy your football. I have to help the staff nurse now. We can talk later.' Reflecting on this incident with her mentor heightened Rachel's awareness of her own discomfort at the time and how she had avoided using the skill of empathetic listening and understanding. She also began to question whether her lack of empathy had hindered her therapeutic relationship with John. She realized that her interventions were aimed at meeting her needs and as such were nurse- rather than person-centred.

Practice exercise

Think back to your most recent clinical placement. Can you identify any situation/ interaction whereby you avoided or limited discussion about the client's feelings? If so:

- What was the situation?
- What strategy did you use to avoid being person/client centred?
- What was the impact of this on the helping relationship?

Learning the skill of empathy

As with most acquired skills, learning how to use the interpersonal skill of empathy and its various components is challenging; even Rogers (1990) admits that he was not always able to achieve these qualities in the relationship. Therefore, to use it effectively will take time, practice and life-long reflective practice. As with all therapeutic communication skills, there are no universal or magical empathetic sentences that will meet all clients' needs or solve their problems. Each client, and therefore each interaction, is unique and will present the mental health nurse with different learning opportunities and challenges. Therefore, in order for real learning and clinical competence to take place, we strongly encourage you to reflect on your use of empathetic listening and understanding, and to be willing to question its effectiveness from a client's perspective. Similar to other therapeutic skills, each nurse or helper will use these skills differently and adapt them according to the situation he/she is in at any particular time.

As with all communication skills, empathy needs to be used with care and genuineness. Before using empathy, the mental health nurse needs to consider the following.

- Usually, empathy-developing statements are tentative, for example 'It sounds as though you are pretty angry at the moment'; 'It feels like you have been sitting on these feelings for a long time'; 'I get a sense that you are very afraid of going back into hospital'.
- Empathy statements should be used sparingly. When over-used, they can sound contrived, false, and not real or genuine.
- It takes time for empathy to develop in a relationship.
- A nurse cannot automatically understand a client's feelings or experiences.
- Non-verbal behaviour should reflect what and how the message is being conveyed verbally.
- Check frequently with the client as to the accuracy of what you are sensing, and be guided by the responses you receive, for example 'I get a sense that you are very afraid of going back into hospital, is that how it feels for you?' Client: 'I am terrified of going back in.'
- Be present for the person and acknowledge that you can never fully understand the client's experience, for example 'I can only imagine how you felt when you were told about your son's suicide.'
- Listen attentively.

Congruence

Congruence or genuineness is another core condition and an important aspect of the helping relationship. This refers to the helper being real or authentic in his/her relationships with clients. Being congruent is a state of being in relation to the client, which comes from the ability to relate to the client as a real person and not to hide behind a uniform, medical jargon or the organization. It means being honest about one's thoughts and feelings; to be oneself without a front or facade. However, it important to be aware that congruence is not the same as self-disclosure. Whereas it is inappropriate and sometimes unwise to be totally self-revealing, the genuine helper is committed to being as open and honest as possible with the other person.

For example, the client has been talking for some time about hearing voices and his frustration with his parents for not believing him. He then stops and asks the nurse, 'You believe me don't you. You can tell my parents that you hear the voices, they will then believe me'. The nurse replies, 'I believe you when you say that you hear voices but I don't hear the voices. We could talk about this with your parents and help them to learn more about your experience of hearing voices. Would this be helpful for you?' Genuineness is usually demonstrated through the helper's verbal and non-verbal communication skills, openness and a commitment to be consistent. Nurses sometimes find it difficult to be congruent with clients, carers, their peers and other members of the health team, for example saying 'yes' when they mean 'no', and as a result are incongruent. See Chapter 8 on assertiveness and communication for further examples.

Unconditional positive regard

Unconditional positive regard (UPC) is acceptance or warm regard for a person, no matter what her/his behaviour, feelings or condition (Rogers, 1961). UPC also means being non-judgemental and non-possessive with regard to the person, and able to demonstrate that acceptance to the client. It does not necessarily mean liking or approving of what everybody does. In fact, there will always be some people whose behaviour you do not approve of or like, but in such situations its working towards separating the person from his/her behaviour and to value the other person as an individual.

So, we have shown the importance of being person-centred as part of your professional helping relationship. We will now consider the characteristics of a professional helping relationship, including setting and maintaining boundaries.

Box 7.1 Characteristics of a professional helping relationship

- **Awareness of self and values:** For example, the use of reflective strategies and a reflective cycle, such as Gibbs's shown in Chapter 3, will help improve your self-awareness.
- **Ability to analyse own feelings:** Again the reflection chapter will provide more detail on how to do this. An example is asking yourself questions such as 'What did I learn exactly from that incident?'
- **Ability to role model:** This requires a fair degree of self-efficacy (explored in more detail in Chapters 4 and 10). An example of this is showing others (modelling) useful examples of communication styles that have a positive effect. You can do this in a therapeutic encounter in several ways, for example if you are working with a client and helping them to relax you may demonstrate how to maximize breathing to bring about state of calm, prior to asking them to demonstrate the exercise to you.
- **Altruism:** To be altruistic in the therapeutic encounter is to show selflessness. You can do this by working through the seven elements of being person-centred and by applying a problem-solving approach (see Chapter 10 for more detail about this).
- **Strong ethical sense:** You can gain this by recognizing some fundamental ethical principles:
  - doing the person no harm, not undertaking duties in which you are not competent
  - being respectful, for example asking the person how they like to be addressed
  - upholding their dignity, for example not being judgemental
  - showing compassion, for example being kind

- acting with integrity, for example not making promises you cannot keep
- being fair and equitable, for example not showing favouritism
- always seeking their consent where possible, asking the person's permission where possible.
- **Responsibility:** You can gain this by remembering that at all times you are acting as a professional and ensuring that you do not consciously, or otherwise, breach your code of conduct. Be mindful of setting clinical boundaries.

Practice exercise

Study the characteristics of a professional helping relationship shown in Box 7.1. Now identify where you have:

1 Strengths
2 Weaknesses
3 Opportunities to improve these characteristics in yourself
4 Threats to you in demonstrating these characteristics.

Setting and maintaining boundaries

As a professional helping relationship, the relationship between the nurse and client or service user is characterized by a code of practice and boundaries (NMC, 2008). A healthy helping relationship is based on trust, which comprises openness and mutual respect. Boundaries define the limits of behaviour between nurse and client. Their function is to protect the client and the nurse. Using the metaphor of a picture, boundaries have been compared to the 'frame' of a picture (Gray, 1994). Therefore, in mental health nursing, the function of boundaries is to contain the client by maintaining the boundary of the clinical work, which in turn can have a positive therapeutic outcome. For example, imagine you are being allocated to a new placement. Allocations have informed you which placement you have been allocated, when you will commence the placement and for how long. You are also informed to contact the unit to find out your shifts. When you phone the ward, the staff nurse is aware of your starting date and informs you of your shifts. As a student mental health nurse, this is a common occurrence throughout your nurse education, which for the most part runs smoothly. Becoming familiar with such practices and, more importantly, the consistency of such practices helps you to feel contained emotionally, conveys a sense of being cared for and allows you to focus on other aspects of your learning, all of which contributes to your ongoing professional and personal learning and development as a mental health nurse.

Now imagine, how you might feel if:

- your name were not on the change of placement list
- you were not informed until the last minute when you were starting and ending your placement
- the ward staff were not expecting you when you arrived on the ward for your placement.

How might you feel? What might you be thinking?

Now imagine how a similar experience might occur in clinical practice involving a client.

The intention of this exercise is to highlight to you the importance of boundaries and their therapeutic value. As a mental health nurse, it is important that you understand and work with boundaries.

Setting boundaries

Setting boundaries at the outset of the therapeutic relationship is important for the client and nurse so that both can make decisions about what is and what is not permitted in the helping relationship. Best practice requires that there should be an explicit verbal working agreement between the nurse and the client from the beginning. While the details of each agreement may vary, clarification and agreement of the requirements, expectations and responsibilities are likely to include the following important issues, as illustrated in the examples below.

- **Confidentiality and the limits of confidentiality.** As a mental health nurse you must respect clients' right to confidentiality and ensure that they are aware of how and why information is shared with those who are providing care. For example, you might reassure a client who is concerned that information concerning his mental health will be disclosed to his family by saying: 'Whatever you say to me will be confidential, that means no information will be shared with your family or anyone else without your consent. However, as you know, I am a member of the MDT and in order for the team to work effectively and for the welfare of clients, we share information about clients with one another. So I will have to tell the team about your suicidal thoughts.'
- **Refusing gifts, favours or hospitality that might be interpreted as an attempt to gain preferential treatment.** For example, a client's relative might want to express her appreciation for the care delivered to her elderly father by inviting you to his 90th birthday party. Whilst very appreciative and flattered to be offered such an invitation, you think about it and decide that it is best to decline the offer by saying: 'Thank you so much for your invitation to your father's

party. It is very kind of you but I am sorry I am unable to attend. I hope your father and your family have a great celebration.'
- **Maintaining clear sexual boundaries at all times with people in your care, their families and carers.** For example, a client whom you have known for several weeks and with whom you have developed a good therapeutic relationship says to you: 'I am being discharged next week. I was wondering if you would like to come out for a drink with me. I just want to say thank you to you.' In response, you might say, 'Thank you for your invitation but I am sorry I cannot meet you for a drink when you are discharged.'

Other issues relating to boundaries may include the following.

- Time boundaries, for example you might negotiate the time boundaries by saying, 'I know that you attend the anxiety management group every Wednesday. I can see you after that, at 4pm until 4.30pm. Does this time suit you?'
- Cancellations of meetings, for example the nurse might say to the service user, 'If you are unable to attend can you please phone me as soon as possible? Also have you got a phone number to contact you if I have to cancel our appointment?'

Sometimes clients may disregard or challenge professional boundaries, either consciously or unconsciously and for many reasons relating to the client's past experiences. It is important that the mental health nurse tries to understand the purpose of the client's behaviour. What is she or he trying to communicate? Working with clients who disregard or challenge professional boundaries can be challenging and the mental health nurse may not know how best to respond. The following are examples of responses that nurses might make to clients in their attempt to restore the boundaries needed.

Maintaining boundaries

Responding to boundary infringements

Boundary infringement	Possible responses
Being asked personal questions that you feel uncomfortable answering, for example:	Politely ignore the question and carry on the conversation. 'I am wondering what has prompted you to ask that question.' *(continued)*

Boundary infringement	Possible responses
Sexualized questions, 'Have you ever been sexually abused?' 'Are you gay?'	'I can see what has prompted you to ask me that question, but this conversation is about you.'
Personal questions, 'Where do you live?'	'That is too personal to answer.'
'How much do you earn?'	'I need to think about that. I will come back to you later about it.'
	'I don't think talking about my experiences is going to be useful to you.'
	It is important to be mindful of your tone and body language, for example tone of voice, facial expression.
	Sometimes letting the client know that you are aware of what s/he is doing, and why they might be doing it. For example, saying the following gently and tentatively may discourage the client from repeating their behaviour: 'I wonder if you are asking me these questions to see whether I will get embarrassed and feel uncomfortable?'
Invading the nurse's personal space, standing too close or physically touching the nurse.	'I would appreciate it if you would stand further back when you speak to me.'
	'Please do not touch my arm.'
	'I want to continue our conversation, but I cannot listen to you if you continue to shout at me.'
Challenging time boundaries, for example always turning up late, going over time by disclosing important information or asking questions at the end of the session.	'I am sorry but we need to end now. I would like you to bring this up next week.'
	'It is important that we start and end at the agreed time.'
	'I have noticed that you tend to ask important questions at the end of the session. I wonder if you want to ask any questions now so that I have plenty of time to answer them.'

The above responses are by no means exhaustive or intended to be prescriptive. We strongly recommend that you practise these responses with your colleagues and mentor, and more importantly reflect on your ability to use such responses, while identifying your strengths and areas for further development.

Having considered the importance of setting and maintaining boundaries in a professional helping relationship and showing you how to demonstrate these in your work, we now move on to the discussing the attributes of effective helpers.

Attributes of effective helpers

Effective helpers show certain attributes that service users appear to appreciate and recognize as being linked strongly to their recovery. These are listed in Box 7.2.

Box 7.2 Attributes of effective helpers (Repper, 2000)

- **Active listeners:** For example, do not interrupt, do pay attention, are non-judgemental, do not give direct advice, clarify anything that is not clear, provide enough time, and do not undermine the person's problem.
- **Respectful**: For example, use a problem-solving approach (see Chapter 10 for an example); do not take sides; are consistent, honest, open and transparent.
- **Tolerant:** For example, do not make judgements that the person might find offensive; make sure that what they say matches their non-verbal behaviour.
- **Trustworthiness:** For example, act on what they promise, but avoid making promises that seem rash and they are unlikely to uphold.
- **Caring:** For example, use a person-centred approach.
- **Friendly:** For example, pay attention to general courtesies; introduce yourself at all times, use small talk (see Chapter 4).
- **Non-judgemental:** For example, do not criticize the person's choices or show disapproval.
- **Sensitive:** For example, demonstrate empathy (see below).
- **Advocate for person they are helping:** For example, whilst enabling the person to remain in control whenever possible, there are times when they will advocate on the person's behalf. You can do this by seeking their permission, being clear as to what expectation they have of you, their desired outcome and what is, and is not, negotiable.

Practice exercise

Sound interpersonal skills are at the heart of professional helping relationships. This exercise is designed to help you assess your interpersonal skills. This may assist you to think about where you have strengths and what issues it may be useful for you to

(*continued*)

work on. Read the following statements. For each statement score yourself from 1, meaning the statement is never true of you, to 5, meaning the statement is always true of you.

1   I introduce myself to the person to whom I am communicating.
2   I avoid the use of swear words.
3   I check the person's name and how they like to be addressed.
4   I agree with the person the goals for the session.
5   I do not interrupt the person when talking with them.
6   I use a consistent tone of voice for the most part.
7   I reflect my understanding of what the person says back to them for clarity.
8   I address issues of confidentiality, being mindful of my code of conduct.
9   I prepare the person for the session coming to an end.
10 I evaluate with the person that they have achieved the goals they set at the beginning of the session.

For those statements where you scored yourself below 3, identify actions you will take to improve these skills.

The interpersonal skills that we looked at in Box 7.2 are some of the core skills required to develop, sustain and end therapeutic encounters. We have shown in Chapter 2 details of how to demonstrate these core skills.

Conclusion

Mental health nursing is essentially a professional helping relationship. A professional helping relationship is different from a personal helping relationship in that mental health nurses have a responsibility to be self-aware, reflect on their ability to analyse their own feelings, model effective interpersonal skills to others, and act selflessly and ethically. Being person-centred in your approach to helping people in your care is likely to enhance your helping capacity. Effective helpers are tolerant, empathetic, sensitive, trustworthy, caring and friendly. They also listen actively and are non-judgemental.

Reflective questions

1   What constitutes a therapeutic helping relationship?
2   What challenges have you experiencing in implementing the core conditions of empathy, congruence and unconditional positive regard?
3   What challenges have you encountered in developing, sustaining and ending professional relationships?
4   Identify factors that can affect the capacity to achieve a helping relationship, from the nurse's perspective and from the client's perspective?

8 | Communicating assertively

Introduction

The ability to speak clearly and directly to clients, carers, peers and other health care workers, whilst being respectful, is an important part of mental health nurses' role. Communicating honestly, succinctly and respectfully is essential for effective nurse–client communication, and the development of good inter- and intra-professional communication and relationships. This chapter will examine the role of assertive communication and its application in mental health practice. We will also identify strategies to build on nurses' ability to become more confident and effective communicators and members of a mental health team.

Learning outcomes

By the end of this chapter, you should be better able to:

1 Describe the components of assertive communication
2 Demonstrate an understanding of how assertive communication can be used to enhance nurse–client communication and professional relationships in clinical practice
3 Use assertive communication in clinical practice

Understanding assertiveness

Assertiveness is an interpersonal behaviour that refers to a person's ability to express his/her beliefs, feelings, needs and opinions without undue anxiety and without denying or devaluing the rights of others (Alberti and Emmons, 1986). It is a way of thinking and behaving that involves open and direct communication while respecting oneself and others. In a nursing context, assertiveness is a communication style that is important to successful relationships for the client, family, the nurse and other health care colleagues (Balzer-Riley, 2000). Its contribution to communication competence and good practice is widely recognized (Hargie and Dickinson, 2004). In fact, in critical or dangerous situations, 'an assertive response can be vital and act as a life-saver for clients' (Larijani et al., 2010, p.894). The following example illustrates the nurse's assertive response as a means of ensuring safe practice.

Clinical scenario

Joan, a newly qualified staff nurse, had begun her first night in charge on the ward. On administering medication with her colleague, she noticed that the dosage of a drug prescribed for a client was higher than the normal range. She decided to check this with the doctor on call before administering the medication. Joan explained the situation to the client and apologized for the inconvenience caused. Her colleague was impatient and said in an abrupt tone, 'The client won't sleep if she doesn't get her medication now. The doctor will not come to the ward for ages.' Joan responded calmly and said, 'I appreciate the inconvenience it is causing the client; however, it is important that the client receives the correct and safe dosage.' An hour later, the doctor arrived and confirmed that the prescribed dosage was within the normal range and was safe to administer. Joan subsequently informed the client and administered the medication. She also informed her colleague, who responded by muttering 'what a fuss for nothing'. Joan considered her response and was satisfied that her response was appropriate and, more importantly, ensured the client's wellbeing.

Choosing to be assertive

Few people, if any, manage to be assertive at all times and in all areas of their lives (McCabe and Timmins, 2006). For many it may be easier to refuse a request, state their needs or express an opinion with their family or friends rather than with their work colleagues. Studies of nurse assertiveness have reported that most nurses feel and act more assertively in situations outside of their work (Fulton, 1997). While there may be many reasons for this, one explanation is that the culture of nursing and the process of professional socialization may decrease nurses' ability to be assertive (Mooney, 2007). Assertiveness is also situation specific – that is, choosing whether to be assertive may be determined by the type of situation presented to the nurse (Rakos, 2003). For example, there may be situations where assertive behaviour may not always be the most appropriate or best response, particularly if there is a high risk of injury to self or others. In such situations, choosing a passive approach may be the best and safest response, as illustrated in the following scenario.

Clinical scenario

James, a qualified nurse, heard raised voices in the dayroom. On entering the room, he observed that there were several family members visiting their elderly father, Mr Green. As he said 'hello', he observed that they were excitable and loud. He wondered whether they had been drinking alcohol. James thought about asking them to leave, as visiting hours had just ended; but given their mood, he considered it best and safer for all concerned to use a passive approach. He approached Mr Green and said 'You have had a busy evening with all your family visiting you. I will come back in 5 minutes and help you to get ready for bed.' One of the family members said loudly, 'I suppose you want us to leave?' James nodded but did not say anything. He returned shortly afterwards to find Mr Green's family leaving the ward and shouting 'goodbye nurse, we're leaving now'. James was relieved they had left without an altercation.

As a concept, assertiveness is not culturally neutral; it has a cultural component, where the person's culture correlates with their level of assertiveness (Yoshioka, 2000). For example, in collectivist cultures, factors such as hierarchy of roles, maintaining harmonious relationships and collective presentation of 'face' are considered important for maintaining good interpersonal relationships (Bond, 1986). Therefore, 'placing emphasis on assertive behaviour, which by definition focuses on the individual, may be culturally inappropriate' (Sully and Dallas, 2005, p.96). In practice, it is important that mental health nurses are mindful of this, particularly when working with clients, families and colleagues from different cultural backgrounds where assertive behaviour may be contrary to the person's cultural mores.

Modes of behaviour

In every interaction, the person responds by using a particular mode of behaviour, which is categorized as follows. For a greater description of all behaviours, see Dickinson (1982).

- Assertiveness
- Passive or submission behaviour
- Manipulative or indirect behaviour
- Aggressive behaviour

Modes of behaviour and OK-ness

Drawing from Eric Berne's theory of transactional analysis and his concept of 'Life Positions', which he called 'OK-ness', each of the four modes of behaviours is underpinned by the person's beliefs about his/her own self-worth and respect, as well as the worth and respect she/he has for others, as illustrated above. For example, assertive behaviour consists of the person's belief that he/she is OK and equally that the other person is also OK; hence the assertive position is 'I'm OK – You're OK' (Berne, 1975).

(continued)

Assertiveness	Passive behaviour
↓	↓
Belief about Self and Others	**Belief about Self and Others**
↓	↓
I'm OK – You're OK	**I'm not OK – You're OK**
Aggressive behaviour	**Manipulative [Indirect] behaviour**
↓	↓
Belief about Self and Others	**Belief about Self and Others**
↓	↓
I'm OK – You're not OK	**I'm OK – You're not OK but I will pretend you're OK**

Source: Adapted from Berne (1975)

Assertiveness: 'I'm OK – You're OK'

This approach involves a way of thinking and being that acknowledges and respects the rights and responsibilities of oneself and others. Assertiveness comprises the following behaviours:

- acknowledging and accepting the strengths and limitations of being human, for example being determined, feeling vulnerable
- using communication that is direct, clear and focused, for example 'I get anxious when I speak to doctors'
- personalizing communication by using 'I' statements, for example 'I feel'; 'I think'; 'I prefer'
- giving constructive criticism, for example 'I feel irritated when you interrupt me'
- seeking opinions of others, for example 'what do you think about ...?'
- endeavouring to negotiate and compromise, for example 'what can we do to solve this?'
- accepting responsibility for behaviour, for example 'I apologize for my impatience this morning'
- setting limits clearly and respectfully, for example 'no, I cannot keep secrets from other health care workers, we work as a team'.

Passive behaviour: I'm not OK – You're OK

This approach is characterized by believing oneself as inferior and not as capable as others, and comprises the following behaviours:

- allowing oneself to be treated with little respect, which is often referred to as being a 'doormat'

- comparing oneself constantly with others, for example 'she is so much better than I am'
- struggling to identify or state needs/wants, for example 'I don't mind, I'll do whatever you think is best'
- finding it difficult to make decisions, for example 'what do you think I should do, you decide'
- fearing upsetting others, apologizes excessively, for example 'I really didn't mean to ...'; 'I am sorry'
- avoiding confrontation, for example will do anything for a quiet life, often says yes when really wants to say no
- using self put-downs, for example 'I'm hopeless at ...'; 'I could never be good at ...'
- dismissing self-worth and value as a person, for example keeps thoughts, opinions, feelings to self
- using long rambling sentences that lack focus and the use of 'I'.

Aggressive behaviour: I'm OK – You're not OK

Aggressive behaviour is competitive, and is characterized by believing that oneself is better than or superior to than others, and comprises the following behaviours:

- finding it difficult to acknowledge mistakes and blames others, for example 'if you hadn't forgotten to remind me about ...'
- using verbal attacks or sarcasm, employing threatening tones and body language, may include finger wagging, raised voice
- not inviting others to share their views, for example 'my view is ... I think ...'
- taking over from others and making decisions with minimal consultation
- using put-downs, for example 'why did you that, I cannot believe you did not know that ...'
- giving heavy handed advice, for example 'you should do it this way'.

Manipulative or indirect behaviour

Manipulative or indirect behaviour may appear subtle, indirect and covert, and comprises the following behaviours:

- lacking genuineness and consistency
- using devious strategies to get what he/she wants, for example making others guilty, 'all I have done for you and now when I ask for one thing'
- using communication that is unclear and dishonest, for example 'I might be able to help you if you support me, you know that I think very highly of you'
- giving mixed messages, for example being nice face-to-face, yet criticizing behind one's back with colleagues
- using sarcasm as a form of indirect or passive aggression

The benefits of being assertive in practice

Much of the nursing literature acknowledges the importance of assertive communication and supports its use for the following reasons (Evans, 2001; Begley and Glacken, 2004; McCartan and Hargie, 2004; Kamile et al., 2006):

- increases job satisfaction
- increases professional opportunities
- equips nurses to empower their clients
- prevents clinical negligence
- increases management skills
- counteracts bullying and stressful situations, and increases self-empowerment
- increases nurses' knowledge and awareness of different methods of responding
- facilitates students to be able to obtain a job, increase their self-confidence and make the transition from student to qualified nurse successfully.

Although assertiveness is advocated as a valuable behaviour, little empirical evidence exists about the frequency and use of assertive behaviours by nurses in the workplace. It is therefore difficult to determine whether nurses are assertive or not (Timmins and McCabe, 2005). Nurses who worked in the areas of mental health, nursing education and nursing administration, however, were identified with more autonomous and independent responsibility and behaviour (Kilkus, 1993).

Factors that affect nurses' level of assertiveness

Research suggests that, in general, nurses are lacking in assertiveness skills (McCartan and Hargie, 2004). Findings suggest that nurses behave in a passive way and are less skilled in disagreeing with other health disciplines, providing constructive criticism and expressing their needs. This lack of assertiveness can contribute to reduced communication efficacy, which in turn can compromise client care (Hargie and Dickinson, 2004). Several reasons have been put forward to explain learners' and qualified mental health nurses' lack of assertiveness. Understanding these factors is important for nurse educators, managers and clinicians. While there is limited research describing the factors that prevent or restrict mental health nurses from being assertive, the following factors have been identified, which militate against the use of assertiveness skills in clinical practice (Burnard, 1992; Poroch and McIntosh, 1995; Farrell, 2001, p.27). Overall, these factors consist of nurses' attitudes, education and the hierarchical organization:

- nurses' belief that assertiveness is closely associated with uncaring behaviour
- nurses' fear of rejection and isolation by colleagues if they use assertive behaviour

- professional socialization, for example the culture of nursing as 'an op-pressed discipline' has encouraged passiveness rather than assertiveness
- nurses' lack of knowledge about their personal and professional rights
- lack of role models for nurses
- hierarchical structure of the health care system, which often discourages nurses and midwives from being assertive
- lack of support from managers.

While the above factors may influence nurses' use of assertiveness skills, it is important to remember that the level of assertiveness may vary from person to person as each interaction is different in personal and professional charac-teristics (Kilkus, 1993). For example, the nurse's gender, age, confidence, life and nursing experience, educational and cultural background might influence his/her level of assertiveness. Interestingly, little information exists about the factors that support the use of assertive skills in clinical practice. Notwith-standing this, nurses and midwives identified responsibility to their clients as a primary motivator of their assertive behaviour (Timmins and McCabe, 2005), particularly in situations where nurses takes on the role of patient advocate, as illustrated in the following clinical scenario.

Clinical scenario

Andrew, a final-year student, attended the multidisciplinary meeting with his mentor, Paul. As part of his learning objectives and with the assistance of his mentor, he agreed to present Joan, a newly admitted client, to the multidisciplinary team. He had reviewed her nursing notes and had spoken to Joan about her progress since her admission. She expressed much concern about her increased weight gain since commencing antidepressants. She requested that her medication be reviewed as soon as possible, and asked Andrew to relay this information to her consultant. At the meeting, Andrew presented the relevant information clearly and succinctly, and answered questions confidently. He stated Joan's concern and her request to review her medication. He was pleased with his ability to present the client's issues clearly and concisely to the team. The consultant thanked Andrew and said 'OK, we must hurry on, it's getting late. Who is the next client?' Andrew was taken by surprise. He felt annoyed and dismissed. He wanted to discuss his client's concern further but he was afraid to challenge the consultant. His mentor, Paul, was also taken aback, and said calmly and confidently to the consultant, 'I know we are running late but I think it's important that Andrew clarifies some issues about his client.' Andrew appreciated his mentor's assistance and proceeded to relay his client's concern about her weight gain and her request to discuss an alternative medication. The consultant appeared irritated, but listened and agreed to see the client after the meeting.

Questions

1   Has this example shown good use of assertiveness or not?
2   What would you do in a similar situation and why?
3   What would you not do in a similar situation and why?

Using assertiveness skills in practice

Assertiveness is a skill that can be increased by education and training (Rakos, 2003). Learning to be assertive involves not only changes in behaviour but also changes in beliefs about oneself. Self-confidence is an important component of being assertive. Mastering assertiveness skills helps to reduce the level of interpersonal conflict, which in turn can reduce the impact of stress on the person (Farrell, 2001). The following skills or techniques are essential to assertive interactions in mental health nursing and are illustrated by various examples from clinical practice:

• saying no
• making requests.

Saying no

In mental health practice, there will be occasions when the nurse will need to say no to clients, family members, peers and other health care workers. For many novice and indeed some experienced nurses, saying no can be anxiety provoking, particularly about the other person's response and fear of being rejected and/or disliked. As a result, nurses often respond by using non-assertive behaviours such as avoidance, being indirect or being aggressive. For example, Agnes asks her colleague Clare if she will swap shifts and work at the weekend. Clare does not want to change her shift but instead of saying no to Agnes, she indirectly refuses the request by giving a rambling and lengthy answer, stating several reasons why she cannot swap shifts, such as 'I am not sure if I can work at the weekend, I would like to help you, but I promised I would baby-sit for my sister. She has a little boy, he is three years old. I promised to baby-sit last week but I was unwell. Do you remember, I couldn't go to your party? My sister never goes out so I want to help her. Did you have a good party? I so wanted to go your party but I was so ill.' Can you imagine how Agnes might be feeling? More than likely, she feels frustrated and says to herself 'all I want is a yes or no'. Sound familiar? Alternatively, an aggressive response might be as follows: 'No I am not swapping my shift for you' (spoken abruptly and loudly), causing the person who made the request to feel embarrassed and dismissed. It is important to remember that although we may feel disappointed when someone refuses a request and says no, if the person says it clearly and respectfully, we are more likely to find it easier to accept, and in fact appreciate the clarity provided by the person's directness.

The principles and practice of saying no

Before the mental health nurse can say 'no' assertively, it is essential that she/he internalize the following beliefs and principles about saying no (Dickinson 1982; Burnard 1992). These include the following.

• **Permission to say no:** Everyone has the right to say no, so just as you have the right to say no to someone, equally the other person has the right to say no to you.

- **Separating the request and the person:** When you say no to someone, it means that you are refusing or rejecting the person's request and not the person, for example 'I don't want to change my shift.'
- **Gut reaction:** Learn to notice your immediate gut response when a request is made. This can be a useful guide as to whether or not you really want to say 'yes' or 'no'. For example, if your gut is getting that sinking feeling as the request is being made, the chances are that you really do not want to agree to the request. It is important to be congruent – that is, be true to yourself and the other person. Be aware of the 'shoulds' or 'musts' that come into your mind and check if they are consistent with what you *really* want. For example, some of the distorted beliefs that might make it more difficult to say no might include 'I should never say no to anyone' or 'I must always be nice.'
- **Taking time:** We often feel that we have to make an instant decision and respond immediately following a request. If you are undecided, take time to make your decision, for example 'I will let you know tomorrow morning if I can change my shift.' It is also important to ensure that you have all the information you need to make the decision, for example 'I need to check if there is transport available at the weekend before I can decide to change my shift.'
- **Avoid waiting:** When you have turned down a request it is common to remain, as a means of offloading any feeling of guilt about the refusal. This can be uncomfortable for both people involved in the refusal. It is best to leave as soon as possible after you have said no, to avoid offloading any feelings of guilt or anger from either person.
- **Saying no:** When you turn down a request, make it very clear that is what you are doing, preferably using the word 'no'. Go straight to the point without any padding, and show you mean it by using assertive body language and tone of voice. For example, 'I have thought about it and no, I do not want to attend the meeting on my own.' The head, neck and shoulder is upright and eye contact maintained while speaking.
- **Broken record:** This involves saying the same thing over and over again, using the same volume and tone until the other person gives up, for example 'No thank you, I don't want a cup of tea', 'No, thank you I don't want a cup of tea.'
- **Using I:** It is best to begin statements using 'I' and make them about yourself and your feelings, thoughts, responses, as opposed to saying 'You', which can sound accusatory. For example, 'I am annoyed with you for constantly changing your shift'; 'I think it's best for everyone concerned that the client does not go home this weekend'; 'I blush and feel nervous when the consultant asks me questions.'
- **No excuses:** When saying no, it is not always necessary to justify your refusal; there may be times however when it is appropriate and helpful to explain your refusal, as illustrated in the following examples: 'No, I cannot allow you to leave the ward at this time. You are on Section 3 MHA, which means that you must remain on the ward for the time being.'

Refusing requests

The following are examples of different situations in which the mental health nurse might need to say no to a client, family member/carer or colleague in clinical practice. They are by no means exhaustive or intended to be prescriptive. It is important to remember that body language must also reflect what is being conveyed verbally.

Requests in clinical practice	Refusing requests in clinical practice
Client: 'Can I go home'?	**Nurse:** 'No, you have to remain on the ward until the doctor assesses you'
Client: 'Can I smoke in the day room?'	**Nurse:** 'No, there is no smoking allowed in the unit'
Client: 'Can I keep my tablets with me?'	**Nurse:** 'No, I have to take them. Medication cannot be kept while you are on the ward. It is the hospital policy'
Client: 'Please don't tell my doctor'	**Nurse:** 'No, I cannot make that promise'
Carer: 'Nurse, would you like a cup of tea?'	**Nurse:** 'No thank you'
Carer: 'Can I give my husband extra medication tonight?'	**Nurse:** 'No, you can only give him what he is prescribed'
Family member: 'What made my son take an overdose?'	**Nurse:** 'I cannot tell you that information without his permission'
Family member: 'You said I could take my son home'	**Nurse:** 'No, that is not what I said'
Doctor: 'I want you to stop Mr X's wife visiting'	**Nurse:** 'No, I cannot stop her from visiting unless she agrees to this'
Consultant: 'Will you witness this ECT consent form'	**Nurse:** 'No, I cannot do that, it is not ethically or legally appropriate'
Social worker: 'Can you take the client back to his hostel today so that he can collect his clothes?'	**Nurse:** 'No I cannot accompany the client, we are short of staff and there is a case review at 11am'
Art therapist: 'Can you stay with the client?'	**Nurse:** 'No, we have discussed this and it was agreed at the team meeting that he could stay on his own'

Making requests

As a mental health nurse, there will be many situations where you will need to make requests to or on behalf of clients, their families and other work colleagues. It is also important to remember that you have the right to make your own wants/needs known to others, particularly concerning your safety and learning, as illustrated by the following examples.

- 'I don't feel confident or competent to carry out a suicide risk assessment'
- 'I don't have enough knowledge about the client's medication to explain it to his father'
- 'I would like to observe this interview'
- 'I would appreciate if you would check whether I have recorded the client's observations correctly'
- 'I would like to learn how to administer an intramuscular injection'

The best chance you have of getting exactly what you want is by asking for it specifically and directly. When you do not ask for what you want, you deny your own needs and importance.

Making requests involves the following principles.

- Decide what it is you want; for some, this may be difficult and unfamiliar. One strategy that might assist you with this is to ask yourself what it is you do not want.
- Once you have decided what you want, the next step is to say it clearly and directly.
- Practise making a clear statement or request without using any unnecessary padding, which is often used when we are anxious. Padding weakens your statement and confuses or irritates the listener.
- Avoid asking indirectly or dropping hints – you run the risk of not being heard or understood and as a result your request may go unheeded.
- State what you want succinctly and with conviction.

Stick to it: after stating your request, you may receive a barrage of abuse, a refusal or even be ignored. This is when you move to the next stage, which is to repeat your statement or request calmly until it is understood and acknowledged by the other person. The purpose of the repetition is to help maintain a steady position without resorting to manipulative or argumentative comments.

Assertive responses

Being assertive also means that the person is able to carry out the following assertive responses (Sully and Dallas, 2005; McCabe and Timmins, 2006). The following illustrates a range of assertive responses and examples of how they might be used in clinical practice.

Assertive responses

Assertive responses	Examples
Express a range of emotions; for example happiness, sadness, anger, fear and guilt	'I am sorry, I feel very sad that you had such terrible experiences of mental health care' 'I am frightened that the client will hit me'
Admit shortcomings; for example self-disclosure about lack of knowledge, skills	'I am not familiar with this antidepressant so I don't know if low blood pressure is a side effect' 'I am a student nurse so I cannot accompany clients off the unit'
Give compliments; for example acknowledging the person's positive characteristic or strengths	'I really liked the way you handled that difficult situation' 'I enjoy working with you, I like the way you respond to clients as people and look for their strengths as opposed to just seeing their diagnosis'
Receive compliments; for example hearing and internalizing positive feedback from another person	'Thank you' 'Thank you for the encouraging feedback'
Initiate and maintain interactions; for example starting and sustaining a conversation with a person	'Hello, my name is Lily. I have just started working on this ward, what is your name?' 'Hi, I notice that you have lots of books in your room, what type of books do you like to read?'
Express an opinion that is unpopular or different from the majority	'I don't think it is appropriate or helpful to label all young female clients as attention seeking or PDs, that is personality disorders' 'I appreciate you are worried about your son, but we cannot use the Mental Health Act to detain him because of his drug addiction'

Assertive responses	Examples
Request behavioural changes by others	'I want you to inform the nursing staff when you want to go to the hospital shop' 'I want you to go to the bathroom if you want to masturbate'
Repetition (broken record) This skill involves using a calm repetition. It helps to stay with the statement or request.	'I want you to leave the ward now. As I said, I want you to leave the ward now. I want you to leave the ward now'

Learning to use assertiveness skills

Learning how to use assertive skills and use them effectively takes time, plenty of practice and motivation, and will present mental health nurses with different learning opportunities and challenges. In order for your ongoing learning to take place, we encourage you to be mindful of the following misunderstanding about assertiveness.

Assertiveness:

- is not about power
- is non-aggressive
- is non-manipulative
- is non-defensive
- does not interfere with other people's freedom to take or not take an assertive stance.

To be assertive does not mean you always get what you want.

Practice exercise: analysis of assertiveness skills

- The aim of this activity is to help you monitor and review your ongoing learning and use of the following assertiveness skills in clinical practice.
- During the next month, try to use each of the assertiveness skills listed below.
- Keep brief notes about your experience of using these skills in clinical practice and answer the questions on the next page.

Assertiveness skills

- Express your emotions in clinical practice
- Ask someone to change his/her behaviour or do something different

- Express an opinion that is unpopular or different from the majority
- Initiate and maintain an interaction
- Receive a compliment
- Give a compliment
- Request something from someone
- Turn down a request – say no
- Admit a shortcoming or limitation

Reflective questions

1 Which of the skills did you find the easiest to use and why?
2 Which of the skills did you find the most difficult and why?
3 Which skill(s) do you want to develop during in your next clinical placement?

Conclusion

Communicating clearly, confidently and respectfully is essential for effective, competent and safe nurse–client communication and practice, as well as good professional relationships. However, learning to be assertive is a challenging, life-long, purposeful, personal and professional activity. For the mental health nurse, it requires a shift in thinking and behaving, and an openness to learn and respect with and from others. As with most learning, acquiring assertiveness skills and developing the ability and confidence to use such skills with clients, peers and other health care colleagues requires time, practice and support from nurse educators, managers and practitioners. Without doubt, assertiveness is often misunderstood and misused by mental health nurses and other health care professionals. It is therefore important to be constantly mindful that assertiveness is a two-way process, which involves not only respecting oneself as a person and mental health practitioner but also respecting the rights of the other person. Although there is some evidence that supports nurses' use of assertiveness in practice, further empirical research is required to explain and support its effectiveness, particularly in the area of mental health nursing.

Reflective questions

1 How would you explain assertiveness to a colleague?
2 What are the benefits of communicating assertively for the mental health nurse? Client? Peers? Work colleagues?
3 Identify three factors that may prevent nurses from using assertive skills in practice.
4 Identify three things that you might consider when saying no a client.

Resolving conflict

Introduction

This chapter examines the nature, sources, causes and consequences of conflict that you may encounter as a mental health nurse, and various communication styles that may help you prevent conflict occurring, or handle it in a therapeutic manner.

Learning outcomes

By the end of this chapter, you will be better able to:

1 Identify the nature, sources, causes and consequences of conflict
2 Describe responses to conflict
3 Examine methods of resolving conflict
4 Practise resolving conflict in a therapeutic manner

The nature, sources, causes and consequences of conflict

Conflict is defined as 'a disagreement through which the parties involved perceive a threat to their needs, interests, or concerns' (University of Wisconsin OHRD, 2006). The NHS Institute for Improvement and Innovation in the UK (NHSIII, 2010) suggests that conflict occurs 'when behaviour is intended to obstruct the achievement of some other person's goals'. Two forms of conflict are identified:

1 hot conflict is where each party involved is keen to meet and resolve the disagreements
2 cold conflict is that where issues are hidden and unresolved (NHSIII, 2010).

As a mental health nurse, you are likely to encounter conflict from several sources:

- threatening disagreements with colleagues
- ambivalence from patients
- resistance to your attempts to help people change, even among those seeking change
- challenging behaviour from patients
- verbal or physical aggression
- unhealthy compliance from patients

Table 9.1 Types of conflict and their presence in mental health nursing

Type	Description	Examples from mental health nursing
Intergroup conflicts	Disagreements in size and complexity between groups	Conflict between nurses and doctors as to the most appropriate form of care
Intragroup conflicts	Disagreements within groups	Conflict between nurse managers and frontline nurses on staffing
Interpersonal conflicts	Disagreements between individuals	Nurse and service user clash over treatment goals
Intrapersonal conflicts	Conflicts with oneself	Having doubts about whether the care you provided was the optimal

Types of conflict

There are four types of conflict (Speakman and Ryals, 2010). Examples of all types of conflict are illustrated in Table 9.1.

Speakman and Ryals (2010, p.190), however, focus their taxonomy of conflict in three key areas.

1 **Affective conflict** is people's perceptions of their relationships with others, for example service user may confuse a professional helping relationship with a mental health nurse as a personal friendship.
2 **Cognitive conflict** concerns the knowledge and understanding people have about a task, for example when working with a service user you instruct them to keep a diary for a week recording things they were doing immediately before bouts of low mood, what we call triggers. Instead of doing this they record how long their low mood lasted.
3 **Process conflict** arises from organizational context, structure, strategy and culture, for example deviating from a care pathway you agreed with colleagues for caring for a service user, leading to harmful inconsistency in care.

Sources of conflict

Sources of conflict vary; some of the key components are shown in Box 9.1.

Box 9.1 Sources of conflict (Pardey, 2007)

- Disagreements between people
- Someone not being up to speed on the fundamentals of a group task
- Complaints or criticism of someone's performance, behaviour or attitude
- Excluding or ignoring others; being silently contemptuous

- A matching of wills, for example a stand-off between colleagues in which neither is willing to concede their position
- Deliberating opposing a request or instruction
- Perceiving someone to be deliberately provocative
- Failing to follow policy
- Taking risks and threatening the security of others
- Aggressive behaviour, for example the use of verbal or physical threats of violence

The sources shown in Box 9.1 provide examples of the different taxonomies of conflict that Speakman and Ryals (2010) report. Consider carefully the list shown in Box 9.1. Now have a go at the following practice exercise.

Practice exercise

Consider the sources of conflict shown in Box 9.1. Alongside each source, identify whether you think it is an example of affective, cognitive or process conflict.

How did you do?

- Affective conflict is 'a matching of wills'
- Cognitive conflict includes 'someone not being up to speed on the fundamentals of a group task'
- Process conflict is indicated by 'failure to follow policy'

Conflict may also occur with the display of certain types of emotional state, for example:

- degrees of emotional intelligence, for example not being sensitive enough (Shih and Susantoi, 2010)
- people showing high levels of expressed emotion, e.g. expressing yourself in a consistently angry tone, or emotional intractability, for example being obstinate (Nair, 2008; Coleman et al., 2009)
- expressing different opinions, beliefs, values (Doucet et al., 2009)
- exercising power and control in situations where the delegation of these may be more appropriate (Liu et al., 2009)
- not being in command of the full and accurate facts of a situation (University of Wisconsin OHRD, 2006)
- using conflicting methods and processes or having alternative goals (Zarankin, 2007).

Consequences of conflict

It is often thought that conflict is inherently dysfunctional. However, a look at the empirical evidence investigating the consequences of conflict challenges

Table 9.2 Consequences of conflict

Negative	Positive
Increased tension	Conflict is identified and resolved
Escalation of conflict	May lead to creativity
Increased stress and frustration	Enhance team performance
Impede decision-making processes	Improve understanding

this view. Speakman and Ryals (2010) review this evidence and show that conflict may have negative and positive consequences, i.e. it may be functional as well as dysfunctional, but this depends largely on how the conflict is perceived. In Table 9.2, we show how conflict can have negative and positive consequences.

There are three common responses to conflict (Webne-Behrman, 1998): emotional, for example getting upset; cognitive, for example forming irrational judgements; physical, for example acts of aggression. These responses are likely to produce conflict, as are the perceptions held by people, including:

- **culture, race and ethnicity** – communicating based on cultural, racial and ethnic stereotypes
- **gender and sexuality** – communication based on stereotypes around gender and sexuality
- **knowledge of situation at hand** – having inadequate knowledge and understanding of the facts of a situation
- **impressions of the messenger** – acting on your view of the messenger, not dealing with the message
- **previous experiences** – of the situation or the person.

Having considered the nature, sources, causes and consequences of conflict, we will now turn our attention to communication strategies that will help resolve conflict. In particular, we will examine methods for preventing conflict, preventing conflict escalating should it occur, containing conflict, managing conflict, building trust and the application of mental health nursing skills towards conflict resolution.

Conflict resolution

On the basis that prevention may be better than cure, we will first consider how you might prevent negative conflict. You are reminded of the distinction between negative and positive conflict as shown in Table 9.2. The remainder of this chapter will focus on negative conflict – that is, conflict that is harmful to the work of individuals, teams and organizations.

Preventing conflict

Earlier we outlined the sequential path that research and ideas about conflict have taken since Pondy's (1966) seminal work on this issue. We showed

Table 9.3 Cooperative versus conflict-provoking communication (Bacal, 1998)

Cooperative communication	Conflict-provoking communication
Active listening, for example not paying attention (see Chapter 1 for more tips on active listening)	Person-centred comments and criticism, for example judging the person, not their behaviour
Empathic responses, for example statements such as 'I imagine that was a difficult situation' (again see Chapter 7 for more tips on how to use empathic responses)	Blaming comments, for example looking for someone to blame instead of seeking to solve the problem
Assertive behaviour, for example expressing an opinion firmly but not aggressively through statements such as 'I disagree with your suggestion'	Inappropriate reassurance and positive thinking, for example being insincere or dishonest so as to appear likeable
Responsiveness, for example changing behaviour that you think is unhealthy	Mistrust statements, for example constantly disbelieving people
	Overreacting, for example taking a heavy-handed approach to a trivial incident
	Showing lack of interest, for example looking bored, such as rolling your eyes, yawning or not listening
	Brush-offs, for example being dismissive
	Threatening language, for example using words or phrases that people may find offensive
	Innuendos, for example insinuating without evidence
	Passive-aggressive behaviour, for example being underhand, not expressing concerns that you have, being silently contemptuous

that conflict was often regarded as an inherent part of organizational culture. There is a limited evidence base on preventing conflict. An exception to this is the work of Robert Bacal. In *Conflict Prevention in the Workplace: Using Cooperative Communication*, Bacal (1998) makes a distinction between cooperative communication – communication that prevents negative conflict – and conflict-provoking communication, that which incites conflict. In Table 9.3, we outline the fundamental distinctions Bacal highlights between cooperative communication and conflict-provoking communication.

Before we turn our attention to how you might improve your cooperative communication, we want you first to reflect upon your potential for conflict-provoking communication. On page 23 of *Conflict Prevention in the Workplace: Using Cooperative Communication*, Bacal provides a detailed self-assessment designed to help you reflect upon your potential for conflict-provoking communication. We have modified some of the verbal and non-verbal examples Bacal associates with conflict-provoking communication that may be relevant to you in your work as a mental health nurse. Read these examples and consider how often you have used them in the last month.

Practice exercise: conflict-provoking communication self-assessment (modified from Bacal, 1998)

Verbal and non-verbal communication	Used in last month
You aren't listening are you?	Yes/No
We tried that before and it didn't work	Yes/No
It's your fault we are in this mess	Yes/No
I can't believe you're making a fuss about this	Yes/No
This is the only way to do it right	Yes/No
Shaking of head while someone is talking	Yes/No
Dramatic behaviour (raising voice, desk pounding)	Yes/No
Raising your eyes	Yes/No
Interrupting someone before they have finished talking	Yes/No
Heavy sighing while someone is talking	Yes/No

Consider your responses to the conflict-provoking self-assessment. What do your responses tell you about your potential to provoke conflict? Do not be concerned if you have used some of these statements or behaviours on occasions in the last month, this is not unusual. However, if you find that you are using conflict-provoking statements and/or behaviours frequently, you may want consider how to switch these for more cooperative communication, for example:

- a focus on problem solving
- highlighting the present and future
- include qualifiers, e.g. 'it might be', 'perhaps'
- admit you could be wrong
- allow people to opt out to save face
- exclude non-responsiveness
- avoid labelling the person
- follow basic communication rules.

(Bacal, 1998, p.39)

In Table 9.4, we have taken five examples of conflict-provoking communication statements, and suggested cooperative communication alternatives. You could use these in a variety of situations, for example when interacting with your mentor if you are a student nurse, or your manager in a clinical situation.

In statement 1, you are signalling your intention to hear their views whilst being able to present your views.

In statement 2, you are opening up the possibility that the present situation may be different and it may be worth revisiting an earlier approach.

In statement 3, you are commenting on the situation, not the person, and offering your help and support to change it.

Table 9.4 Replacing conflict-provoking statements with cooperative communication alternatives

Conflict-provoking statements	Cooperative communication alternatives
1 'You aren't listening are you?'	'It would help me if I could finish, then I'd like to hear your views'
2 'We tried that before and it didn't work'	'I remember trying this before and it didn't work for me, what might be different now that may make it worth trying again?'
3 'It's your fault we are in this mess'	'This situation feels messy, what might we do to change it?'
4 'I can't believe you're making a fuss about this'	'I'm not sure I understand your reaction, could you explain it a bit more?'
5 'This is the only way to do it right'	'Have you tried this approach? I've found it helpful in the past'

In statement 4, you recognize that you are lacking an understanding and seeking further information.

In statement 5, you are offering help based upon previous successes with the suggested approach.

Practice exercise

Consider the different communications styles shown in Table 9.3. Identify encounters from your work where these styles were apparent and reflect on the outcomes that arose from these encounters.

Bacal's work focuses on communication styles that prevent or foment conflict. Other authors focus on organizational climates linked to conflict. For example, Borcher (1999) distinguishes between defensive and supportive climates. The latter is of interest in preventing conflict. The features of a supportive climate include:

- people feeling able to present ideas and opinions
- a willingness to listen to such ideas
- a focus on problem solving
- open and honest communication
- empathy, and equality – that is, seeking opinions and ideas.

The source of the evidence behind Borcher's ideas is not clear. However, there is a strong evidence base behind the concept of ward atmosphere (see Moos, 1997, for example) and Borcher's notion of the supportive climate taps in to similar issues in that a supportive climate is likely to lead to better working relationships between people. In your work, you may be leading teams. Fostering a supportive climate may prevent conflict in your teams.

Containing and preventing conflict from escalating

Despite attempts to prevent conflict using the methods proposed above, negative conflict is a common feature of organizational life. We will now turn our attention to managing conflict. A useful starting point is taking steps to prevent the conflict escalating. You can prevent conflict escalating by identifying:

- the type of conflict (see Table 9.1)
- what are the important underlying influences?
- what is the conflict really about?
- where the conflict may be heading?
- how can you stop it?
- what needs to happen immediately?

(NHS III, 2010)

Central to preventing the conflict escalating is considering how to contain the conflict. You can contain conflict by:

- recognizing your own strengths and weaknesses
- listening to and trying to understand the person with whom you are in conflict
- asking questions to develop a fuller understanding
- looking for a solution(s) that satisfies all parties.

Sound interpersonal and problem-solving skills are required to contain and prevent conflict escalating. The key skills are: listening actively (see Chapter 1), being solution-focused (see Chapter 10), knowledge and understanding of the nature, sources and causes of conflict (see above), and a range of facilitative and authoritative interventions (see Table 9.7 below).

Managing conflict

Here are some general tips on managing conflict.

- **Remain calm:** It is important to show that you are in control of the situation. If you appear anxious and agitated people may have little faith in your ability to manage the conflict, as a result, you may exacerbate the conflict.
- **Show empathy and concern:** Avoid appearing insincere and take managing the conflict seriously. Look interested by paying attention to what people are saying. Show that you understand people's concerns and the emotional impact it has on them. Statements such as 'that must have been a difficult situation to find yourself in' will demonstrate empathy.
- **Do not make rash promises:** Think carefully before you commit yourself to solutions. Consider the pros and cons of any potential solution, seek advice and support from people in whose judgement you have confidence. Check out your ideas with them. Rash promises that you cannot keep will also foment the conflict and could lose you people's trust irredeemably.
- **Treat people with respect:** Show that you are solution-focused by using the problem-solving approach we discussed in Chapter 10. Give all parties

Table 9.5 Handling conflict (NHS III, 2010)

Do	Don't
Ensure that issues are fully outlined	Use a public place
Acknowledge emotions and communication styles	Leave the discussion open
Ensure comfortable environment	Finish people's sentences
Set a time frame	Use jargon
Establish good rapport	Constantly interrupt
Use names/titles as appropriate	Be distracted
Seek to cool tempers	Distort the truth
Show that something can be done about the conflict	Use inappropriate humour

in the conflict equal space to share their grievances. Do not take sides; take positions and act in a consistent manner to all parties. It is also important to be honest, open and transparent and keep all parties informed of what you are doing to manage the conflict.

In managing conflict, we recommend a person-centred approach. Being person-centred means recognizing that people's behaviour is communicating information about their thoughts, feelings and beliefs. It is central to the positive nursing approach we advocate in Chapter 2, and will take account of the values and cultural aspects of communication, as well as drawing upon the best possible evidence to handling conflict. In Table 9.5, we show some helpful 'dos' and don'ts' when handling conflict (NHS III, 2010).

Pardey (2007) identifies seven factors that promote conflict resolution. In Table 9.6, we describe these factors and give you an opportunity to assess your conflict resolution skills and make an action plan to develop your skills in resolving conflict.

Practice exercise: developing skills in conflict resolution

1 Consider the seven factors that are thought to promote conflict resolution, shown in Table 9.6.
2 For each factor shown in the second column, assess your level of skill by allocating a score between 1 and 5, where 1 indicates little skill and 5 indicates a high degree of skill.
3 Based on your skill level for each factor, in column 3 assess the degree of change you may need to develop your skill by putting TW for tweak where you require minor improvement, TU for turn if you require a moderate improvement or TR for transform if you require major improvement.
4 In the final column, outline specific actions you will take to improve your skill for each factor. Some examples are given to assist you.

This practice exercise is especially helpful when trying to help resolve conflict where you have a responsibility for leading a team and managing staff. It starts by asking you to rate your skill level, assess the degree of

Table 9.6 Conflict resolution skills

Conflict resolution skill	Score 1–5	Assessment of required improvement: tweak (TW) score of 4–5 turn (TU) score of 3 transform (TR) score of 1–2	Specific action you will take to improve skill
Example: Listen actively	4	TW	I will interrupt people less when listening to them
1 Example: Equipping yourself with the facts of a situation	3	TU	I will ask all parties to give me their views on the situation
2 Distinguishing between the problem and the person	1	TR	I will judge the person's behaviour and not them, by using statements such as 'I found your behaviour unacceptable in that situation'
3 Clarity in your communication style			
4 Maintaining contact between parties in conflict			
5 Looking for the needs and interests that lie behind fixed positions			
6 Making it easy for the parties to be constructive			
7 Developing your ability to look at the conflict from outside			

improvement you think you need and ask you to identify specific actions to improve your skill where required. We now want you to consider a situation that is commonly found in the workplace.

Conflict resolution scenario

You are the leader of a community mental health team. James and Jane are valuable members of the team, but they do not get on and are forever undermining each other. For example, when Jane tries to contribute in meetings, James always undermines her by dismissing her suggestions out of hand. It is now affecting the operation of the team and your ability to work with them. From what you have learnt so far about resolving conflict between others, describe how you might resolve this conflict between James and Jane. For example, a good start may be to ask James and Jane to self-assess the extent of their conflict-provoking communication style and their cooperative communication styles. Once they have self-assessed their styles, ask them to rate each other's styles. Use the results of these assessments to formulate a plan to help James and Jane to manage their conflict.

Resolving conflict through effective interpersonal communication

In Table 2.3 of Chapter 2, we demonstrated the features of developing, maintaining and ending therapeutic encounters, and the role that active listening and empathy play in this process. Throughout the book, we have shown how active listening and empathy link to effective communication. Bacal (1998) recognizes the importance of active listening and empathy in preventing conflict as part of cooperative communication. However, he also advocates the value of responsiveness, 'speaking or acting in a way that responds to others' needs in a clear way' (Bacal, 1998, p.66). Your skills in listening actively or responding empathically show that you understand a person's needs or issues; responding shows that you are prepared to act on this understanding.

Five steps to being responsive are:

1   assess the underlying needs of others
2   check out your assessment with them for accuracy
3   offer to help them meet their needs
4   help them as promised
5   check that your help has had the desired effect.

(Bacal, 1998)

High degrees of personal self-awareness coupled with specific actions are recommended when trying to resolve conflict; these include the following:

- **Knowing and taking care of yourself:** For example, using Gibb's model shown in Chapter 3 will help improve developing your level of self-awareness. In addition, you can assess the extent that you use cooperative communications styles or conflict-provoking styles using Bacal's self-assessment tool shown above.
- **Clarifying personal needs threatened by conflict:** For example, reflect carefully on what it is specifically about the conflict that is threatening to you. Ask yourself questions such as 'What am I feeling?' 'What might be my contribution to the conflict?' 'What do I think about it?' Consider whether you are experiencing any physical symptoms because of the conflict.

- **Identifying a safe place for negotiation:** For example, try to avoid using locations where people may feel tense, too cold, too hot, noisy, crowded, lacking privacy. Select a setting that people are comfortable in, use small talk (see Chapter 4) to warm up the situation, ensure people are sitting comfortably and avoid places that may seem to prefer one party to another – that is, use a neutral location.
- **Asserting your needs clearly and specifically:** For example, be clear to own contributions you make using statements that begin with 'I', such as 'I would like to suggest . . .', avoid speaking about yourself in the third person or using statements such as 'some people think . . .'; be specific, identify who these people are. Do not be vague about what you are saying; use statements such as 'I do not agree with your assessment of the situation.'
- **Approaching problem solving flexibly:** For example, do not take a fixed position or be obstinate. Show in what you say and how you behave that you are willing to consider many options to resolve the conflict, use a problem-solving approach (see Chapter 10), do not take sides or take positions, and be willing to compromise.
- **Managing impasses with calm, patience and respect:** For example, remain optimistic, between sessions stay in contact with each party, do not appear anxious, agitated or harassed, allow all parties time to make a contribution, show verbal/non-verbal congruity, i.e. ensure what you say matches your behaviour, do not make promises you cannot keep.
- **Building an agreement that works in the long term:** For example, avoid rushing into decisions that may have short-term value but not work in the long term. Identify quick wins, i.e. immediate solutions to take the heat out of a situation, medium-term goals and long-term goals. Always check out whether agreed solutions are having the desired effect and be prepared to renegotiate solutions that are not working.

(University of Wisconsin, 2006)

The following clinical scenario illustrates how Joe, a third-year student, managed to resolve the interpersonal conflict with his mentor.

Clinical scenario

Joe is a third-year student enjoying working in the admission ward. It is his favourite placement. He had a good relationship with the service users, nursing staff and members of the MDT. Unfortunately, due to sickness, his mentor, Sarah, was unable to continue her role. Joe was subsequently allocated a new mentor, Terry. Although Joe understood the reasons for changing mentor, he was disappointed and anxious that he and Terry would work well together. He liked Terry but he knew he could be impatient and very critical, particularly of student nurses. Joe discussed his fears with his partner and peers, who reassured him that he would be fine, after all 'he always got on well with his mentors'. Over the coming weeks, Joe and Terry worked closely together. Terry was a conscientious mentor and spent time providing feedback to Joe. Whilst Joe appreciated Terry's input, he became increasingly fearful and frustrated with Terry since his feedback always focused on his areas of weakness. At first Joe tried to ignore his feelings of anxiety and anger and told himself that 'it will get better with time'. However, Joe became aware that he wanted to avoid going to work. This concerned him and he decided that he needed to resolve this conflict before the situation deteriorated further. Joe knew that he needed to talk to Terry, but he was afraid that Terry might become more critical and give him a bad ward report. He reflected on his fears and discussed the incident with his peers. He recalled telling a client recently to be assertive and confront his critical employer. Joe decided that he needed 'to practise what he preached' and express his fears to Terry. He thought and practised what he might say and how he might say it. The next day, Joe spoke to Terry and said, 'I appreciate your help and guidance as my mentor, you have given me a lot of time. I know that I learn best when I get feedback on my strengths – that is, what I am doing right and what I could do better. I know you mean well, but your feedback is sometimes very critical and that makes me nervous and then I lose my confidence.' Terry listened and said nothing for a few minutes. Joe felt scared and thought to himself 'He is going to fail my clinical assessment.' Terry then said, 'OK, thank you Joe for telling me this. I didn't tell you your strengths because I thought you knew them. I will try to work on this in future.' Over the coming weeks, Joe noticed that Terry tried to be more encouraging and constructive when giving feedback. Joe also began to take more responsibility by asking Terry directly 'what did I do well in . . .'

Resolving conflicts with service users

Earlier in the chapter, we alluded to different interventions that you might use to resolve difficulties arising from interpersonal conflict. One such approach is that advocated by Heron (2001). Heron's approach is humanistic and identifies six categories of intervention that you might find helpful in resolving conflict. See Chapter 5 for further coverage. In Table 9.7, we show how to apply Heron's model to an interpersonal conflict with a service user, Tony.

Clinical scenario

Tony is a 30-year-old man for whom you are caring on an acute ward and who is detained under section 3 of the Mental Health Act. Conflict with Tony arises from his repeated absconding from the ward due to being anxious around strangers. Because Tony is detained under the Mental Health Act, he is not permitted to leave the ward unless his Responsible Clinician approves this. Tony, however, believes that he should be able to leave the ward whenever he wants, and repeatedly absconds. As a result, the police bring him back to the ward and this makes him angry. This is causing conflict between you and Tony. Table 9.7 shows how you can resolve this conflict using Heron's model.

Table 9.7 The use of Heron's Six Category Intervention Analysis to resolve conflict

Intervention	Description	Phrases to consider using to resolve conflict with Tony
Prescriptive	Being directive	'I want you to negotiate leave with me instead of absconding'
Informative	Providing knowledge or information	'If you abscond from the ward the police will be called to bring you back'
Confronting	Raising awareness of effect of behaviour	'I notice that you abscond mostly during lunch when we are very busy, as a result we have to take time away from other patients to deal with your leaving the ward. Are you aware of this effect?'
Supportive	Confirming validity of someone's feelings	'It must be hard to be restricted on the ward'
Catalytic	Enabling the person to discover their own solutions	'What might help you deal with your anxiety other than absconding?'
Cathartic	Helping the person share their feelings	'It's understandable to feel anxious around strangers'

In evaluating the effect of Heron's approach, Morrissey (2009) suggests checking, rechecking and, if necessary, modifying the approach (demonstrated above) with Tony to check its success. This can also be done alone, with a colleague, with your mentor or in clinical supervision.

For the final sections of this chapter, we want to examine the role of trust in resolving conflict and end the chapter by looking at what works in conflict resolution as reported by published empirical evidence.

The role of trust in conflict resolution

Trust plays an important role in resolving conflict and is likely (NHS Institute for Innovation and Improvement [NHS III, 2008], trust is likely if you demonstrate to others that you care about people, and you are competent and capable, as shown in Figure 9.1.

The key to building and keeping trust is:

• acting on what you say
• not making promises that can't be kept
• active listening
• understanding people's needs
• keeping their best interests in mind.

To a large degree, the issues involved in developing and keeping people's trust are similar to the concept of responsiveness (see above) that Bacal (1998) reports.

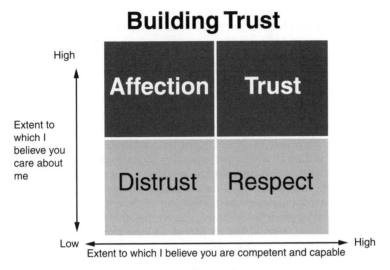

Figure 9.1 The link between trust and care, and competence and capability

There is evidence showing the link between trust and conflict resolution. This evidence shows:

- trust was an important factor linked to strong team identification and reduced conflict (Han and Harms, 2010)
- to be effective teams must conceive of themselves as a discrete unit and create and maintain trust within each team member; failure to do either could have detrimental effects on team performance (Han and Harms, 2010)
- conflict had a deleterious effect on trust (Ayoko and Pekerti, 2008).

What works in resolving conflict?

We have examined the nature, sources, causes and consequences of conflict, analysed communication styles that may prevent, exacerbate and resolve conflict, and considered how you can prevent conflict occurring or handle it in a therapeutic manner. In line with the general approach in this book, we have drawn upon multiple sources of evidence, from that of expert practitioners, our own expertise in using and teaching these methods to nursing, health and social care students, and published empirical evidence. We want to end the chapter by looking at key points from the latter in resolving conflict. These are summarized below.

- A high level of self-efficacy (belief in your ability) helps resolve conflict (Desivilya and Eizen, 2005).
- Strong group identity improves conflict resolution (Desivilya and Eizen, 2005).
- First-line management support moderates the impact of conflict (Thomas et al., 2005).

- Among Chinese managers, embarrassing colleagues and teaching moral lessons was instrumental in conflict management; among American managers, hostility and vengefulness were seen as impediments to conflict resolution (Doucet et al., 2009).
- Aggression is likely to exacerbate conflict (Coleman et al., 2009).

Conclusion

Mental health nurses are likely to encounter conflict in their day-to-day work; some of this conflict is welcomed as it may improve performance and communication; much of it is unwelcome because it may increase tension, stress and frustration, and lead to poorer outcomes for patients. Conflict may be prevented by a cooperative communication approach. When conflict arises, there are several approaches to minimize its negative impact and bring it to healthy conclusion. Mental health nurses seeking to resolve conflict should prevent it escalating by the following.

- Use person-centred issue-based approaches.
- Seek to build trust in their relations with patients and colleagues.
- Be prepared to use a variety of authoritative or facilitative interventions.
- Be mindful of the cross-cultural differences in conflict management.
- Seek to raise their levels of self-efficacy, and promote cohesion and strong identity in teams in which they work.

Reflective questions

1 Which one of the following is an example of intragroup conflict?
   - Conflict between nurse managers and frontline nurses on staffing
   - Conflict between nurses and doctors as to the most appropriate form of care
   - Nurse and service user clash over treatment goals
   - Having doubts about whether the care you provided was the optimal
2 What are five examples of cooperative communication that may minimize conflict?
3 How might you use Pardey's seven skills in resolving conflict in your work as a mental health nurse?
4 Why is trust important in resolving conflict?

10 Solution-focused interventions in mental health nursing

Introduction

This chapter is concerned with solution-focused interventions in mental health nursing. Solution-focused interventions are those that are highly structured, have an agreed ending that is communicated to the client at the outset, involve cognitive and behavioural components, and focus on helping clients seek their own solutions. We will concentrate on three particular approaches: solution-focused brief approaches, cognitive behavioural approaches and problem-solving interventions. Our aim is to examine solution-focused approaches, consider the similarities and differences between each approach, evaluate the evidence base for each approach and consider the clinical application of each approach, to help you improve your communication skills when working with people in a professional helping relationship.

Learning outcomes

By the end of this chapter, you should be better able to:

1 Describe solution-focused approaches
2 Identify the similarities and differences between each approach
3 Evaluate the evidence base for each approach
4 Consider the clinical application of each approach to help you improve your communication skills when working with people in a professional helping relationship

---

Solution-focused interventions

Solution-focused brief therapy (SFBT)

As the name suggests, SFBT, which arose from the work of de Shazer and colleagues at the Brief Family Therapy Centre in Milwaukee, USA (de Shazer et al., 1986), emphasizes the notion of *solution building* by looking at a person's existing resources and future hopes. A typical programme of SFBT lasts for around five sessions. De Shazer and colleagues found that when clients exhibited problem behaviour, there were inconsistencies in this behaviour – what they called exceptions, i.e. clients exhibiting healthy as well as unhealthy behaviours. It was within these exceptions that solutions to the behaviour were found.

In common with other solution-focused interventions, SFBT is also goal-orientated, i.e. the clearer a client's goals are, the greater the chance of these goals being achieved. Within the identification of goals lie the client's future hopes. SFBT may be used as a discrete intervention on its own, or with other interventions (Iveson, 2002). SFBT has been used with a range of client presentations including depression (Sundstrom, 1993), eating disorders (O'Connell, 1998), substance misuse (Dolan, 1991) and sexual abuse (Dolan, 1991).

In Box 10.1 we describe the characteristics of SFBT (de Shazer and Berg, 1997; Gingerich and Eisengart, 2000).

Box 10.1 The characteristics of SFBT

- The therapist's use of the 'miracle' question (see Table 10.1 below)
- Use of scaling questions, for example asking the client 'On a scale of 1–10, can you rate your problem-solving skills in general'
- A consulting break, for example allowing time off for the client to work on set tasks
- Giving the client compliments, for example praising them when they are making progress
- Assignment of homework tasks to work on between sessions, for example client agrees to go for a ten-minute walk every day
- Exploring strengths and solutions, for example the client identifies existing strengths and solutions they have used in the past to deal with a current problem
- Goal setting, for example agreeing with the client the objectives of the session
- Exploring exceptions to the problem, for example asking the client to identify occasions when the problem did not exist

---

The first session in an SFBT intervention appears crucial in understanding the client's concerns, and setting goals (future hopes) to address these concerns. Table 10.1 outlines what Iveson (2002) calls the key tasks of the first session of SFBT. We have adapted this to show how you can use this approach in any therapeutic encounter, and we provide examples of questions that you may use in this encounter.

Iveson suggests a useful metric that you can use to help the person assess his/her current state, and their ideal state. This is shown in Figure 10.1.

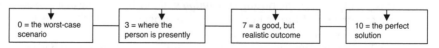

Figure 10.1 The Scale Framework (Iveson, 2002)

Table 10.1 Key tasks during the first session of solution-focused interventions (adapted from Iveson, 2002)

Mental health nurse's task	Questions that may help the mental health nurse achieve his/her task
Explore what the person is hoping to achieve from the encounter	'What are you hoping to achieve from our session today?'
Explore what life would be like if the person realized their hopes	'Imagine you wake up tomorrow and you have realized all your hopes; what do you think would be different?' This is regarded as the 'miracle' question
Explore what the person is doing now, or has done before, to realize their hopes	'Think of a time when you have realized your hopes in the past. What did you do then?'
Explore what might be different if the person took a small step towards realizing their hopes	'What things would you, or those close to you, notice if you realized some of your hopes?'

To make use of the scale ask the client to identify where they are on it, i.e. the point of sufficient satisfaction to them. The scale is used to define:

- the client's goals
- what they are already doing to achieve these goals
- what their next step might be.

Using the miracle question is likely to help the client describe the perfect solution. Therefore, for a client with incapacitating depression, the perfect solution might be a life completely free of depressive symptoms. A good and realistic outcome for the same client is managing the depressive symptoms so that they can get on with their lives. Where the client is now involves exploring with them what they have done that has helped them arrive at this point or what they have done to prevent a worsening of their problem. It is best not to explore in too much detail the worst-case scenario, but it is worth bearing in mind that, for depressed person, this could be a life of overwhelming depression with little remission from their symptoms.

Practice exercise: using a solution-focused communication style

You are working in a community mental health team and one of your clients is Mary. Mary has been a long-standing client of the team, but has made little progress with a succession of colleagues. You have been asked to work with Mary as it is thought she may benefit from a solution-focused approach. All you know of Mary is that she has a long history of cutting her arms when distressed. From what you have read so far about solution-focused communication, describe how you might help Mary overcome her distress without cutting her arms. Pay particular attention to the aims and characteristics of solution-focused styles, where the emphasis lies when communicating using this approach, and the key tasks and questions in your initial assessment of Mary.

The efficacy and effectiveness of solution-focused brief therapy

Gopfert (2002), while acknowledging the value of SBFT, questions its lack of explanatory power, and the lack of systematic evaluation of its efficacy and effectiveness. Previous published work on SFBT tended to report clinical studies, many of which eschewed systematic evaluation. However, since 2002, there has been a significant increase in research testing the efficacy and effectiveness of SFBT. The key points from this research are:

- SBFT was significantly better than no intervention or treatment as usual, suggesting practical significance (Corcoran and Pillai, 2007)
- SFBT produced small, positive effects when compared with alternative interventions, but only the effects of SBFT on internalizing behaviour problems such as depression, anxiety of self-concept were significant (Kim, 2008)
- SFBT appeared to improve substance use, self-esteem and behaviour problems in schoolchildren (Kim and Franklin, 2009).

These results show that SFBT has promise in producing therapeutic outcomes that may be of relevance to mental health nurses and the people for whom they care. Mental health nurses could incorporate the characteristics of SFBT into a solution-focused communication style with relative ease, which may add to their repertoire of therapeutic communication skills.

Cognitive behavioural approaches

Cognitive behavioural approaches derive from the theories of behavioural psychologists such as Skinner in the 1950s and cognitive theorists such as Beck in the 1960s. These theories have been combined into a therapeutic intervention, which is now referred to as cognitive behaviour therapy (CBT). CBT is a psychological intervention for various mental and behavioural disorders that also incorporates components of other therapeutic approaches (e.g. rational emotive therapy, problem-solving interventions, coping skills training). Gelder (1989) states that the development of CBT was due to:

- recognition that thoughts and feelings are central to many mental health problems
- CBT filling a gap between behavioural and psychodynamic therapies
- CBT being scientific and more amenable to evaluation in clinical trials.

Meichenbaum (1997) identified three particular features of CBT:

1 links between thoughts, feelings and behaviour, and the resultant consequences, social context and physiological processes
2 short-term (< 20 sessions) highly structured intervention
3 sensitive to the role of warmth, empathy, emotional attunement, acceptance, providing hope, bolstering client's self-efficacy and nurturing a therapeutic alliance.

In CBT, a client is helped to recognize patterns of distorted thinking and dysfunctional behaviour and through systematic discussion is helped to develop behavioural assignments to evaluate and modify the distorted thoughts and dysfunctional behaviour. The process of CBT will largely be influenced by the nature of the client's presenting problems. Table 10.2 shows features common to most applications of CBT.

CBT is now used in the treatment of a wide range of mental, behavioural and physical disorders, including:

- the management of persistent symptoms of schizophrenia resistant to medication (Sensky et al., 2000)
- anxiety (Clark, 1989)
- obsessive-compulsive disorders (Salkovskis and Kirk, 1989)
- depression (Fennell, 1989)
- eating disorders (Fairbairn and Cooper, 1989)
- medication concordance (compliance) (Kemp et al., 1996)
- HIV/AIDS (Molassiotis et al., 2002)
- chronic fatigue syndrome (Price and Cooper, 2000).

The efficacy and effectiveness of cognitive behavioural approaches

CBT has been evaluated through numerous well-designed studies across a range of mental health and other health problems. For example, it is shown to be:

- superior to befriending (having a buddy or friend to help), especially in the long term in clients with persistent symptoms of schizophrenia resistant to medication (Sensky et al., 2000)
- better than standard care alone in reducing relapse rates in people living with schizophrenia (Jones et al., 2000)
- beneficial in improving physical functioning in adult outpatients with chronic fatigue syndrome, when compared with relaxation or medical management (Price and Cooper, 2000).
- better than peer support and counselling or no formal intervention in Chinese people symptomatic with HIV living in Hong Kong (Molassiotis et al., 2002)
- beneficial for anxiety disorders, phobias, obsessive compulsive disorder, post traumatic stress disorder, chronic pain and depression (O'Carroll, 2006).

There is now an established evidence base for many CBT approaches. The Oxford Guide to Low Intensity CBT Interventions (Bennett-Levy et al., 2010) reports on the many applications of these approaches and the evidence base supporting these interventions. Many of the interventions can be used with ease by mental health nurses in their day-to-day practice with minimal additional training. The final part of this chapter will examine problem-solving interventions.

Table 10.2 Common features of CBT

Assessment	Treatment	Evaluation
Behavioural interview, e.g. an interview to establish the nature and extent of the problem behaviour and its effect on the client's life	Cognitive restructuring – this involves helping the client to change negative thoughts into more realistic ones	Anxiety outcomes, e.g. measuring the client's anxiety levels by questionnaire, pulse, blood pressure or taking a blood test to detect adrenaline levels
Self-monitoring, e.g. asking the client to keep a diary noting when the behaviour occurs and what might have triggered it	Cognitive re-appraisal, e.g. asking the client to re-assess the conclusions they draw from certain incidents. If the client fails a driving test and they conclude that they are a failure, asking them to identify things in which they have succeeded to counteract the negative conclusion	Behavioural outcomes, e.g. measuring differences in the client's behaviour such as dealing with a feared object instead of avoiding it
Self-report, e.g. asking the client to complete a rating scale to assess the level of depression; the Beck Depression Inventory can be used for this	Coping skills, e.g. suggesting ways in which the client can improve their coping skills; you can teach them how to relax by breathing deeply and slowly if anxious, instead of overeating	Compliance levels, e.g. measuring the client's adherence to treatment
Information from others, e.g. asking other people involved in the client's life what they think	Problem solving (see Table 10.4 below)	Client's perception of success, e.g. asking the client for their views on how successful the treatment was for them
Direct observation, e.g. noting what you observe about the client's behaviour during the interview	Behavioural activation, e.g. helping the client to identify things that give them pleasure and helping them to do more of these things	Level of coping skills, e.g. measuring how well the client copes with everyday issues that were once a problem for them, such as when a client with claustrophobia takes a lift instead of using stairs
Physiological measures, e.g. if the client is anxious, checking their pulse and blood pressure	Guided self-help, e.g. helping the client identify self-help manuals and guiding them through using these on their own	Physiological changes, e.g. changes in heart rate
	Exposure, e.g. used in treating phobias where the client is exposed gradually to a feared object and helped to manage their fear	
	Response prevention, e.g. often used with exposure whereby when the client is exposed to a feared object they are disallowed from using safety behaviours to avoid the object	

Using cognitive behavioural approaches in mental health nursing

This section focuses on how you can use aspects of cognitive behavioural approaches in your communication with people for whom you care. In Table 2.3 we outlined the core attitudes, values and skills required in developing, maintaining and ending therapeutic encounters. These are also important in using cognitive behavioural approaches in your everyday practice. We recommend you refer to Chapters 2 and 7.

We will now focus on four different aspects of cognitive behaviour approaches:

1 the five areas approach
2 behavioural activation,
3 cognitive restructuring
4 problem solving.

The five areas approach

The five areas model is an approach to assessment using cognitive behavioural principles that Chris Williams and colleagues (Williams and Chellingsworth, 2010) at the University of Glasgow developed. The five areas approach adheres to the traditional cognitive behavioural approaches of showing how thoughts, feelings and behaviours interact in developing and sustaining dysfunctional anxiety and mood disorders such as depression. It is an approach that can be incorporated with relative ease into the day-to-day practice of mental health nursing. Figure 10.2 illustrates the five areas approach.

We shall demonstrate how you can use this approach with someone for whom you are caring.

Practice exercise

Susan is a 38-year-old mother of two young children who has been referred to your mental health team by her GP who believes she is anxious. She has been allocated to your caseload. You are conducting as assessment interview with Susan, during which you use the five areas approach. The following illustrates how you can use this approach.

1   Ask Susan to identify a specific and typical situation where she has recently felt highly anxious. She reports a sudden phone call from her husband to say he must remain at work and requesting Susan to pick up the children from school. Susan has not done this for some time and recalls feeling highly anxious when she did this because she felt the other parents were talking about her in a negative manner.
2   Having identified the specific situation, ask Susan to record the altered thinking associated with this situation. For example, this might include 'I thought I was a bad mother.'

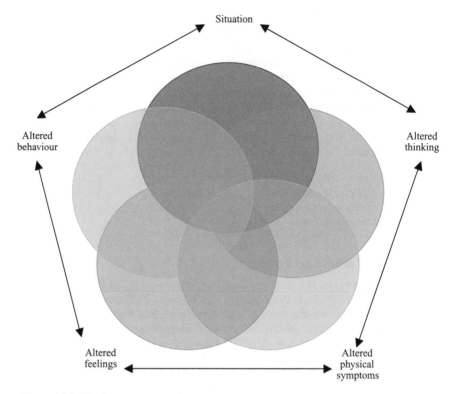

Figure 10.2 The five areas approach to assessment

3 Ask Susan to record physical symptoms associated with the situation. These may include feeling hot, flushed, sweaty and panicky.
4 Ask Susan to identify altered feelings associated with the situation. For example, these may include feeling anxious.
5 Finally, ask Susan to record altered behaviour linked to the situation. This may include refusing to leave the house because of the anxiety.

There are several benefits to using the five areas approach.

- It helps you capture important information about a client's thoughts, feelings and physical symptoms, and how these influence behaviour.
- It gives you a structure to your assessment.
- It involves the client actively.

Having used the five areas approach in your assessment, you may use some cognitive behavioural approaches as a treatment. We describe four such approaches below, starting with behavioural activation.

Table 10.3 Six steps in using behavioural activation (from Richards and Whyte, 2009)

Six steps	Mental health nursing activities
Step 1: Explain BA, e.g. BA is an intervention that helps people re-create everyday routines and increase activities that give them pleasure	Key things to communicate to David are the relationship between physiological, cognitive and behavioural symptoms, how avoidance sustains low mood, and how routine, pleasurable and meaningful activities can change things
Step 2: Identify routine, pleasurable and necessary activities	Ask David to identify things that he would normally do if he were not depressed
Step 3: Make a hierarchy of routine, pleasurable and necessary activities	Ask David to rank the activities identified in step 2 in order of importance: low, medium and high priority
Step 4: Plan some routine, pleasurable and necessary activities	Help David plan routine, pleasurable and meaningful activities starting with the lowest ranked initially. This could form the basis of a week of planned activities that David can record in the form of a diary
Step 5: Implement BA exercises, i.e. participating in the routine, pleasurable activities	Help David carry out the planned activities and ask him to make a list of the activities he does, for example taking the dog for a walk, visiting a friend, listening to music
Step 6: Review progress	Review progress with David by asking him to list those activities he managed to complete

Behavioural activation (BA)

BA is a structured psychological intervention that is often used as part of CBT, but has an increasingly strong evidence base when used on its own (Richards, 2010). The effectiveness of BA derives from it usefulness in targeting avoidance in people with depression (Richards and Whyte, 2009). Essentially, BA is an intervention that helps people re-create everyday routines and increase activities that give them pleasure. Mental health nurses are well placed to use BA in day-to-day work. Table 10.3 outlines the six steps of BA and we show you how to use these steps when working with people in your care, using David as an example. David is a young man living with depression who you have taken on to your caseload in your role as a nurse in an early intervention team.

BA focuses mostly on re-discovering *behaviours*, the everyday routine and pleasurable activities that have given people satisfaction, but that have been dormant as a result of depression. BA is method of working with people on behavioural change. When people are depressed they often express automatic thoughts that are unhelpful, intrusive and, although they are real to the person expressing them, are generally irrational and likely to perpetuate their low mood. Cognitive restructuring is an approach that you can use to help people to modify automatic thoughts by assisting them to recognize, scrutinize and confront them. We will now explain how to incorporate cognitive restructuring into your work as a mental health nurse.

Cognitive restructuring

Richards and Whyte (2009) identify three stages to cognitive restructuring. We shall demonstrate how you can use these stages with David, to whom we referred in our BA exercise.

Clinical scenario

- **Stage 1 – Recognizing thoughts:** Ask David to identify a situation in which he felt a particular emotion. Such a situation may include failing a driving test, a job interview or a relationship breakdown. Ask him to rate the emotion on a scale of 0–10 with 0 being the weakest emotion and 10 being the strongest. Following this, ask David to write down the automatic thoughts associated with the situation, e.g. failing a driving test could lead to the automatic thought of being a failure as a person. Help him to pin down the most salient thought, the so-called 'hot thought', and the one causing the greatest distress. Finally, ask David to identify the strength of his belief in the hot thought from 0, little belief, to 10, the strongest belief.
- **Stage 2 – Search for the evidence:** Ask David to choose an automatic thought to work on, usually the 'hottest thought' with a rating of at least 6 out of 10. For this thought, ask David to write down the evidence for and against this thought. For example, David's hottest thought is 'I am a failure as a person, that's why I failed my driving test.' Ask him to write down what evidence leads him to this conclusion. Now ask him to write down evidence to challenge this conclusion. For example, 'I failed my driving test because I did not prepare enough. I have succeeded at things for which I have prepared.' This approach allows for a more balanced assessment of the conclusion.
- **Stage 3 – Restructuring thoughts:** Help David to re-examine the automatic thoughts in light of the evidence identified in stage 2, write down new thoughts and consider the feelings associated with the new thoughts. For example, having re-examined the evidence, David is likely to put the driving test failure into context in light of his success at other things and will thus feel better. Then ask David to rate his strength of belief in each new thought from 0–10. Finally, help David to recognize how his feelings may change after having identified new thoughts.

  Having considered the value of helping people to modify automatic thoughts by assisting them to recognize, scrutinize, confront and challenge these thoughts and thus recover from depression, we now turn our attention to what is a common-sense approach to dealing with overwhelming problems: problem-solving interventions.

Problem-solving interventions (PSI)

PSI are brief psychological approaches that involve helping clients identify specific problems, arrive at helpful solutions, implement the solutions and evaluate the effect of these solutions (Mynors-Wallace and Lau, 2010). PSI are recommended by the National Institute for Health and Clinical Excellence (NICE) for the treatment of minor to moderate depression. PSI are underpinned by a view that everyday problems contribute to people's symptoms, therefore if the problem can be tackled, and hopefully resolved, the symptoms will reduce or disappear. There are seven stages to PSI.

- **Stage 1:** This is where you explain what is meant by PSI, e.g. tell the client that PSI help people identify specific problems, list helpful solutions, use these solutions and assess their impact.
- **Stage 2:** This involves identifying specific problems in a clear and concise manner, for example 'I sleep for three hours each night.'
- **Stage 3:** This is where the person identifies all potentially helpful solutions to the problems identified in stage 2, for example sleeping for eight hours each night.
- **Stage 4:** At this stage the person is ask to prioritize all potential solutions and select the most helpful.
- **Stage 5:** Here, the person plans how to implement the solutions, for example avoiding drinking coffee before bed.
- **Stage 6:** At this stage, the person implements the chosen solutions.
- **Stage 7:** During this stage, the person assesses how successful the solutions have been.

Mental health nurses can use PSI easily and, in Table 10.4, we show examples of how you can help people in your care use PSI to help them recover. The stages shown in Table 10.4 can be used in brief encounters with the person or as part of a longer session. If you learn quickly how to use this approach with people in general, you will equip yourself with a valuable set of therapeutic tools that have been shown consistently to help people overcome everyday problems that threaten to incapacitate them. A basic PSI session takes around 30 minutes to complete. Three to four sessions should suffice.

The efficacy and effectiveness of PSI

PSI is sometimes referred to as problem-solving therapy (PST). There is a strong evidence base demonstrating the efficacy and effectiveness of PSI across a variety of problems and cultural groups. This evidence base shows PSI:

- was better than usual treatment (Gellis and Kenaley, 2008)
- had a positive effect in people with emotional disorders, self-harm and physical health problems (Mynors-Wallis and Lau, 2010).

Table 10.4 Applying problem-solving interventions in mental health nursing (Richards and Whyte, 2009; Mynors-Wallace and Lau, 2010)

Stage of PSI and features of stage	Role of mental health nurse
Stage 1: Explanation of PSI	Explain the rationale and evidence base (see below) for using PSI, e.g. show how everyday problems can contribute to symptoms and how PSI can help resolve problems and tackle symptoms
Stage 2: Identify and define problem(s)	For each problem identified, break it down into specific parts, e.g. lack of interest in everyday issues can be broken down into: **what** kinds of everyday issues **when** these occur **where** they occur and **who** may be involved It might help to rank the problems in order of most to least troublesome
Stage 3: identify specific solutions	Help person recognize all possible solutions and the resources they can bring to the solutions
Stage 4: Choose a solution for each problem	At this stage, you can help the person select what they think will be the most appropriate solution for each problem. Helping them recognize their resources to deal with solutions is important to ensure they do not fail because of choosing an inappropriate solution. For example 'what do you think will help you to go for a walk each day?', 'who could help you to get out of the house every day?'
Stage 5: Planning the implementation of chosen solutions	Help the person make sensible plans to implement chosen solutions, for example: **what** exactly will they do? **when** exactly will they do this? **where** will they do it and with **whom**?
Stage 6: Implement chosen solutions	The person implements the solution and you ask them to keep a record of their progress
Stage 7: Evaluation	Here, you help the person reflect on their progress towards solving the problems; reinforce where there has been progress

Conclusion

There is a strong evidence base showing the efficacy and effectiveness of solution-focused interventions. Most mental health nurses, some with little additional education, can use many of the interventions shown in this chapter with relative ease. The solution-focused interventions presented in this chapter require strong partnership working between you and the people for whom you care professionally. They are interventions that enable people to identify, and use systematically, their own resources towards their own recovery.

Reflective questions

1 What are the four key tasks for nurses using SFBT and what questions can mental health nurses use to achieve these tasks?
2 How can you use the five areas approach to assessment in your clinical work?
3 Why might you use the six stages of BA in your clinical work?
4 What examples from each of the approaches described in this chapter help you to improve your communication skills when working with people in a professional helping relationship?

 # Motivational interviewing in mental health nursing practice

Introduction

This chapter introduces motivational interviewing (MI) and a step-by-step guide to how to use the principles of MI in practice. In particular, we will focus on distilling what is MI, the theory underpinning MI approaches, the phases of MI and examining in detail how mental health nurses can apply MI skills in routine practice.

Learning outcomes

By the end of this chapter, you should be better able to:

1 Describe MI
2 Describe the theory behind MI
3 Discuss how mental health nurses can use MI in routine practice

---

What is motivational interviewing?

Mental health nursing often involves helping people change from being over-whelmed by mental distress, to a position where they recover to lead lives that are meaningful and satisfying to them. People seeking mental health care are often looking to change aspects of their lives. However, people seeking change are often ambivalent, and may lack the will, ability or readiness to change (Hettema et al., 2005). MI is a person-centred, but directive, therapeutic intervention designed to help people improve their readiness to change (Miller and Rollnick, 2002). MI has its practical origins in humanistic approaches to therapy based upon the work of Carl Rogers (1961). Box 11.1 shows the key features of MI.

Box 11.1 Features of motivational interviewing

- A counselling method which is a form of therapy
- Designed specifically to evoke health-related behaviour change

- Person-centred, i.e. the focus is on the person seeking help, not the nurse providing help
- Directive in momentum, i.e. the purpose of MI is directed towards arriving at a solution helpful to the service user
- Relationship building, i.e. developing a sound therapeutic relationship is a core component of MI (see Chapter 2 on how to do this)
- Uses cognitive and behavioural processes to assess and improve stages of change, i.e. MI is about helping people recognize how unhelpful thoughts might shape behaviour, challenging these thoughts and thus changing the behaviour
- Emphasizes the resolution of immobilizing ambivalence, i.e. the nurse challenges the service user's ambivalence about change
- Does not evoke arguments against change, instead promotes change
- Seeks to elicit person's own reasons for change – that is, help the person identify their reasons for change
- Uses reflective listening in directive manner – that is, listen carefully to what the person is saying and reflect themes back to them

Self-motivational statements

It is important to listen for and reinforce increases in five self-motivational areas:

1 self-esteem, for example how the person feels about themselves
2 concern, for example concern for change
3 competence, for example ability to change
4 knowledge of problems and strategies
5 desire for change.

When applying MI at an early stage of the therapeutic encounter, be careful to establish an atmosphere of trust and acceptance, allow the person to explore his/her problems, allow the person to do most of the talking, listen carefully and ask open-ended questions (see Chapter 1). In Box 11.2, we outline some ways in which you can develop skills in using MI in everyday therapeutic encounters.

Box 11.2 Developing skills in using MI in everyday therapeutic encounters

Explanatory questions

'You say heroin helps you cope – tell me a little more. What does it help you cope with?'

(continued)

'You say you have worries about using crack. Can you tell me what worries you?'

Reflections

Making a guess as to what the person means by reflecting it back to them for confirmation or clarity, 'it sounds as if you are not certain about ... '

Information is often coded; hear the words and understand the meaning. Check out with the client if you are unsure, for example 'can I just check that I have understood you correctly? You say that ... '

Return the client's reflection as a statement not a question, for example 'so you're more anxious when around certain friends than others ... '

Avoid asking **'why'** questions; why questions can give the impression that you are expressing moral disapproval. Instead of asking 'why did you do that?' say, 'Tell me the reasons behind that action.'

The five principles of MI

There are five fundamental principles of MI:

1 expressing empathy
2 developing dissonance
3 avoiding arguments
4 rolling with resistance
5 supporting self-efficacy.

The following are examples of how to apply these principles in your work as a mental health nurse.

- **Expressing empathy:** Make statements that show you understand the impact of the client's problems on their life, e.g. 'That must have been traumatic for you.'
- **Developing dissonance:** When developing dissonance we recommend using an antecedent-behaviour-consequence approach (ABC). The ABC approach consists of:
    - **antecedent:** identifying the immediate event that precedes a given behaviour
    - **behaviour:** identifying how a person responds generally to a given behaviour
    - **consequence:** identifying what occurs as a result of the given behaviour.

Phillips and Callaghan (2009) outline how this approach works in practice with a person using illicit substances. See below how the ABC approach is used with Paul, who struggles to contain his aggressive impulses and whom you encounter while working on an acute inpatient ward.

- **Avoiding arguments:** Do not get into a war of attrition with the client.
- **Rolling with resistance:** If the client states that they do not want to work with your suggestions, ask them to identify actions they think might work and help them prioritize a list of what actions to take first.
- **Supporting self-efficacy:** Raise the client's belief in their ability to help themselves by asking them to make a list of actions that have helped them successfully in the past, trying these actions again and, where successful, praising the client for their efforts.

Practice exercise

Paul was admitted to your ward three days ago. His behaviour since admission has been erratic, characterized by bouts of verbal and physical aggression towards staff and other patients, and moments where he is calm and affable. The following practice example shows you how to demonstrate skills in caring for Paul using the ABC approach to help him understand what his aggressive behaviour represents.

Antecedent	Behaviour	Consequence
Ask Paul to list immediate triggers for his aggression, e.g. feeling neglected, being bored.	For each of the triggers ask Paul to list how he generally responds to these triggers, e.g. he assaults staff and other patients.	Paul is restrained, and restrictions are imposed on his time out of the ward.

Using the ABC approach to help Paul manage his aggressive impulses to avoid the negative consequences, you may want to consider the following alternative.

Antecedent	Behaviour	Consequence
Paul identifies that he is feeling neglected and is bored.	Paul asks you for some therapeutic time to discuss how to deal with his feelings of neglect and boredom.	Paul gets 30 minutes of therapeutic time with you. You agree that he can have time out from the ward to take a walk. He thus avoids being restrained and having restrictions placed upon him; i.e. his behaviour now has positive consequences.

(continued)

- It is important that you make clients aware of the possible consequences of continuing with the behaviour that they regard as problematic, for example for someone who misuses substances you can say: 'Have you thought of what might happen if you continue to inject harmful drugs using needles shared with others?'
- Your role is to help the client highlight the discrepancy between what they want to achieve, and their current behaviour, for example 'You say that it is your goal to avoid getting infected with HIV, yet you are still injecting drugs using needles that you share with other drug users and this is a major source of HIV infection.'
- You can also help the client note how changing their behaviour will help them achieve desired goals, for example 'If you inhaled the heroin instead of injecting it, you will avoid the risk of HIV infection though this route.'
- It is crucial that you show change is possible, e.g. share your successes with previous clients, and that you instil hope by remaining positive about the client's ability to change.

Applying the three phases of MI in mental health nursing

There are three phases of MI:

1 the eliciting phase
2 the information phase
3 the negotiation phase.

The *eliciting phase* is characterized by assessing readiness to change. For example, the use of a Readiness to Change questionnaire or ruler will help establish how ready the person is to change the unhelpful behaviour. For example, when using the Readiness Ruler, you ask the person to rate on a score of 1–10 how ready they are to change. For people seeking your help to change their substance misuse pattern, you may ask them three specific questions:

1 How important is it to change their substance misuse pattern?
2 How confident are they that they can change their substance misuse pattern?
3 How realistic is it that they will avoid substance misuse in the long term?

In the *information* phase, you seek the client's views as to their goals for changing unhelpful behaviour. For example, in relation to substance misuse you may pose the question: 'What is your goal for the substance you misuse?' You may want to anchor the responses as:

- 'not using at all'
- 'cutting down'
- 'continuing to use or undecided'.

In the negotiation phase, you work with the person to agree a plan for how change may occur. For example, you may ask the client to consider: what actions they have taken in the past to change their substance misuse; what worked well, less well or what did not work at all.

For those actions that had some previous success, ask the client to consider what made them successful and what they can learn from these to change current behaviour.

Practice exercise

To help you understand how to apply the three phases of MI, identify a friend with whom to try this exercise. First, ask your friend to identify any aspect of their lifestyle they want to change. This may be changing to a healthier diet, taking more exercise or spending more time on leisure pursuits. Once they agree on a lifestyle change, ask your friend:

1 To rate on a scale of 1–10 how ready they are to change, 1 being not at all ready, 10 being maximum readiness. If they score 5 or above they are sufficiently ready to change. If they are ready to change:
2 To rate on a score of 1–5 how important is the change to them, 1 being of no importance, 5 being of huge importance. A score of 3 or above suggests they think it is important to change. Now:
3 To rate from 1–5 how confident they feel to make the change, 1 being not all confident, 5 being extremely confident. A score of 3 or above suggests they are sufficiently confident in their ability to change. Finally:
4 To rate from 1–5 how realistic it is that they will avoid their previous lifestyle if they make the change to a different lifestyle, 1 being little likelihood, 5 being highly likely. A score of 2 or below suggests there is little likelihood they will revert to their previous lifestyle. Now:
5 To identify what is their main goal in changing their diet/taking more exercise/ spending more time on cultural pursuits? Now:
6 To make a list of things they can do to change their diet/take more exercise/spend more time in cultural pursuits. It may help to remind them of things that worked for them in the past when trying to change these aspects of their behaviour. Now:
7 To rank the list of things with the most important being at the top of the list and the least important being at the bottom of the list.
8 To work through the list in order of priority.

The three phases of MI work alongside other aspects of MI that we will now consider. We will start with considering a theory behind using MI, and show you how you can use this theory in communicating effectively using MI.

Applying MI theory to communicating using MI

MI has its roots in the Transtheoretical Model of Change, or TTM (Prochaska and Marcus, 1994; Callaghan et al., 2010). The TTM has four related concepts considered central to behavioural change. These are stage of change, self-efficacy, decisional balance and process of change. These will now be explained in relation to exercise.

Stages of change are the client's current state of behaviour. An example of the stages in relation to exercise is as follows.

1 Precontemplation – not even thinking about exercising.
2 Contemplation – seriously considering exercising.
3 Preparation – making plans to change by joining a gym.
4 Action – exercising regularly at the gym but for fewer than six months.
5 Maintenance – exercising regularly for more than six months.
6 Relapse – reverting to not exercising regularly.

The TTM proposes that individuals progress through a series of stages before they achieve a sustained change in the behaviour. When assessing people's stage of change the mental health nurse has several tasks to consider, which are shown in Box 11.3.

Box 11.3 Stages of change and the mental health nurse's tasks

- Pre-contemplation – ask questions about the client's readiness to change
- Contemplation – help person to identify reasons for change
- Preparation – help person determine best course of action, for example joining an exercise group, a gym or using stairs instead of lifts
- Action – help person make a plan to change, for example help negotiate access to facilities, accompany them on brisk walks, enrol them on your unit's exercise activities
- Maintenance – help person identify and use strategies to prevent relapse, for example ask client to keep a diary of activities and how they feel; reinforce the positive benefits they identify
- Relapse – help person revisit reasons for change as in contemplation

---

Self-efficacy is the client's belief that they have the confidence to change their exercise behaviour, even under adverse conditions like being too tired. You can assess the client's self-efficacy levels by asking five simple questions (Callaghan et al., 2010). These are:

Ask the client how confident they feel – from not at all confident scoring 1, moderately confident, scoring 3 or extremely confident scoring 5 – about exercising even when tired, in a bad mood, when the weather is poor, when they don't have time and even when on holiday.

Individuals with high self-efficacy should feel confident that they could exercise even when faced with barriers such as tiredness, time pressure or a bad mood. Exercise self-efficacy should increase as individuals move through the stages of change towards maintenance.

Practice exercise

Consider the five questions designed to assess self-efficacy for exercising. Answer each question and calculate your own self-efficacy score. A total score close to 5 suggests that you are low in self-efficacy, a total score close to 25 means that you are high in self-efficacy. Consider your total score and reflect what your score might mean for how you can help improve a client's self-efficacy.

Decisional balance is the client's assessment of the pros and cons of exercising. You can assess the client's decisional balance by using the questionnaire in Figure 11.1 designed for this purpose (Callaghan et al., 2010).

		Not at all important		Moderately important		Extremely important
1	I would have more energy for my family and friends if I exercised regularly.	1	2	3	4	5
2	Regular exercise would help me relieve tension.	1	2	3	4	5
3	I think I would be too tired to study after exercising.	1	2	3	4	5
4	I would feel more confident if I exercised regularly.	1	2	3	4	5
5	I would sleep better if I exercised regularly.	1	2	3	4	5
6	I would feel good about myself if I kept my commitment to exercise regularly.	1	2	3	4	5
7	I would find it difficult to find an exercise I enjoy that is not affected by bad weather.	1	2	3	4	5
8	I would like my body better if I exercised regularly.	1	2	3	4	5
9	It would be easier for me to perform routine physical tasks if I exercised regularly.	1	2	3	4	5
10	I would feel less stressed if I exercised regularly.	1	2	3	4	5
11	I feel uncomfortable when I exercise because I get out of breath and my heart beats faster.	1	2	3	4	5
12	I would feel more comfortable with my body if I exercised regularly.	1	2	3	4	5

Figure 11.1 Decisional Balance Questionnaire (*continued*)

	Not at all important		Moderately important		Extremely important
13 Regular exercise would take too much of my time.	1	2	3	4	5
14 Regular exercise would help me have a more positive outlook on life.	1	2	3	4	5
15 I would have less time for my family and friends if I exercised regularly.	1	2	3	4	5
16 At the end of the day, I am too exhausted to exercise.	1	2	3	4	5

Figure 11.1 Decisional Balance Questionnaire (*continued*)

Typically, individuals who exercise have a positive decisional balance in that the positive beliefs about exercise outweigh the negative beliefs. In contrast, the decisional balance of sedentary individuals is generally negative (Callaghan et al., 2010). In addition, as individuals progress through the stages, a systematic shift in decisional balance should occur. Specifically, pros should increase when individuals move from pre-contemplation to contemplation. In contrast, cons should decline progressively in the move from contemplation to action and maintenance.

Practice exercise

Select a client with whom you are working and have a discussion about exercise. Using the decision balance questionnaire as a guide, discuss with the client the pros and cons of exercising. From their responses to these questions, list five pros and five cons of exercising for this client.

The final part of the TTM is the processes of change. Processes of change are any activity that the client does to modify their mood, behaviour, cognition or relationships. An example of the processes and how you can use them when communicating with clients about exercise are shown in Box 11.4.

Box 11.4 Examples of process of change

Name of process	Description	Ask the client to identify
1. Consciousness raising	Increasing knowledge about the benefits of exercise	Some benefits of exercising
2. Dramatic relief	Reacting to warnings about the risks of not exercising	Their typical reaction to warnings about not exercising

Name of process	Description	Ask the client to identify
3. Environmental re-evaluation	Caring about consequences to others of not exercising	How they feel not exercising affects how others see them
4. Self-re-evaluation	Comprehending the benefits of exercise	How they might *feel* if they exercised more
5. Social liberation	Increasing healthy opportunities to exercise	Opportunities to exercise near where they live
6. Self-liberation	Committing yourself to exercise	How committed they are to exercising
7. Helping relationships	Enlisting social support to help you exercise more	Who they can turn to for help to exercise more, e.g. a friend who is a regular exerciser
8. Counter-conditioning	Substituting alternatives	How they can take advantage of opportunities to exercise more, e.g. asking GP for some exercise on prescription vouchers
9. Reinforcement management	Rewarding yourself	How they can reward themselves for exercising more
10. Stimulus control	Reminding yourself to exercise	Reminders to exercise, e.g. leaving reminders around the house or asking the gym to text a reminder

These ten processes can be categorized into two broad classes, namely Experiential and Behavioural. Experiential processes cover individuals' awareness of how exercise may help them, and their feelings about exercising. Processes 1–5 are examples of experiential processes. Behavioural processes are things that individuals do to help them exercise, such as rewarding themselves when they exercise, having friends who encourage them to exercise and placing things around the house that will remind them to exercise. Processes 6–10 are examples of behavioural processes. People generally use different processes during particular stages of change. For example, individuals in the 'lower' stages, namely Precontemplation, Contemplation and Preparation, generally use more experiential and fewer behavioural processes than people in the more active stages, namely Action and Maintenance. In contrast, those in

Action and Maintenance generally use more behavioural and fewer experiential processes (Callaghan et al., 2010).

In the final part of this chapter, we want to consider the evidence for the efficacy and effectiveness of MI in mental health care.

Evidence-based MI

There have been many studies published testing the effect of MI. We will report the key results of several important studies.

When compared with no treatment or placebos, i.e. dummy treatment, MI produced:

- a 56% reduction in problem drinking and a 51% reduction in substance misuse (Burke et al., 2003)
- a 59% improvement on general health and mental health outcomes (Hettema et al., 2005)
- improvements in psychotic symptoms and satisfaction with medication (Maneesakorn et al., 2007)
- improved the participants' self-esteem, quality of life, depression and social support (Callaghan et al., 2010).

In summary, health care professionals who use MI are more likely to:

- extract more change talk
- decrease resistance levels from clients
- increase the likelihood that clients will change their behaviour in a positive direction.

Therefore, mental health nurses seeking to help people change are likely to succeed if they adopt MI. The strength of their commitment to helping people change is important to whether change in clients actually occurs.

Conclusion

MI has the potential to help you in your everyday therapeutic encounters with people seeking your professional help. Many of these encounters may involve helping people change an aspect of their behaviour that they find unhelpful or troubling, or that affects negatively their day-to-day life. By assessing people's readiness to change, seeking information on desired goals for change, negotiating strategies to help the person change behaviour to achieve these goals and applying the five principles of MI, you are enhancing your therapeutic encounters. Consequently, your communication becomes more person-centred and humanistic, and it is facilitating positive change that will help people in your care achieve meaningful and satisfying lives – an important step in their recovery from overwhelming mental distress.

Reflective questions

1 What is the mental health nurse's role in using the ABC approach to reduce incidents of violence on a mental health unit?
2 When using the Readiness to Change Ruler in working with a person seeking to change their substance misuse, identify three specific questions that may help them understand their readiness to change.
3 At each of the six stages of change, what is the key task for mental health nurses?
4 What are the five principles of MI? What is the rationale behind each principle? In addition, what mental health nursing skills can you use to apply these principles in practice?

Conclusion

Reflective questions

References

Agar, M. (1994) The intercultural frame. *International Journal of Intercultural Relations* 18(2), 221–237.

Alberti, R.E. and Emmons, M.E. (1986) *Your Perfect Right: A Guide to Assertive Behaviour*, 4th edn. St Lois Obispo: Impact Publishers.

Alexander, J. and Bowers, L. (2004) Acute psychiatric ward rules: a review of the literature. *Journal of Psychiatric and Mental Health Nursing* 11, 623–631.

Allot, P. (2005) *Celebrating Cultural Diversity: Developing Cultural Capability*. NIMHE, University of Wolverhampton.

Anthony, P. and Crawford, P. (2000) Service user involvement in care planning: the mental health nurse's perspective. *Journal of Psychiatric and Mental Health Nursing* 7, 425–434.

Arnold, E. and Underman Boggs, K. (2003) *Interpersonal Relationships Professional Communication Skills for Nurses*, 4th edn. London: WB Saunders.

Atkins, S. and Murphy, C. (1993) Reflection: a review of the literature. *Journal of Advanced Nursing* 18(8), 1188–1192.

Ayoko, O.B. and Pekerti, A.A. (2008) The mediating and moderating effects of conflict and communication openness on workplace trust. *International Journal of Conflict Management* 19(4), 297–308.

Bacal, R. (1998) *Conflict Prevention in the Workplace: Using Cooperative Communication*. Winnipeg, Mb: Bacal Associates.

Balzer-Riley, J. (2000) *Communication in Nursing*, 4th edn. St Louis: Mosby.

Barker, P. (2003) *Psychiatric and Mental Health Nursing, The Craft of Caring*. London: Arnold.

Barker, P. and Buchanan-Barker, P. (2005) *The Tidal Model: A Guide for Mental Health Professionals*. London: Routledge.

Barret-Lennard, G. (1981) Dimensions of therapeutic responses as causal factors in therapeutic change. *Psychological Monographs General and Applied* 76, 1–36.

Bee, P., Playle, J., Lovell, K., Barnes, P., Gray, R. and Keeley, P. (2007) Service users' views and expectations of mental health nurses: a systematic review of empirical research. *International Journal of Nursing Studies* 45(3), 442–457.

Begley, C.M. and Glacken, M. (2004) Irish nursing students' changing levels of assertiveness during their pre-registration programme, *Nurse Education Today* 24, 501–510.

Benner, P. (2001) *From Novice to Expert. Excellence and Power in Clinical Nursing Practice*. Upper Saddle River, NJ: Prentice Hall.

Bennett-Levy, J., Richards, D., Farrand, P. et al. (2010) *Oxford Guide to Low Intensity CBT Interventions*. Oxford: Oxford University Press.

Benson, A. and Minghella, E. (1995) Developing reflective practice in mental health nursing through critical incident analysis. *Journal of Advanced Nursing* 21, 205–213.

Berne, E. (1975) *What Do You Say After You Say Hello?* New York: Grove Press.

Bhui, K., Stansfeld, S., Hull, S. and Priebe, S. (2003) Ethnic variations in pathways to and use of specialist mental health services in the UK. *British Journal of Psychiatry* 182, 105–116.

Biggs, J. (1999) What the student does: teaching for enhanced learning. *Higher Education Research and Development* 18(1), 57–74.

Bischoff, A., Bovier, P.A., Isah, R., Francoise, G., Ariel, E. and Louis, L. (2003) Language barriers between nurses and asylum seekers: their impact on symptom reporting and referral. *Social Science and Medicine* 57, 503–512.

Bond, M.H. (Ed.) (1986) *The Psychology of the Chinese People*. Hong Kong: Oxford University Press.

Bonham, P. (2004) *Communication as a Mental Health Carer*. Cheltenham: Nelson Thornes.

Borchers, T. (1999) Conflict in groups. Accessed from http://www.abacon.com/ commstudies/groups/conflict.htmlon 24 October 2010.

Boud, D., Keogh, R. and Walker, D. (1985) What is reflection in learning? In: Boud, D., Keogh, R. and Walker, R. (eds) *Reflection: Turning Experience into Learning*, pp. 7–17. London: Kogan Page.

Bowers, L., Brennan, G., Winship, G. and Theodoridou, C. (2009) *Talking with Acutely Psychotic People: communication skills for nurses and others spending time with people who are very mentally ill*. London: City University.

Boyd, E.M. and Fales, A.W. (1983) Reflective learning: key to learning from experience. *Journal of Humanistic Psychology* 23(2), 99–117.

Bricker, D., Glat, M. and Stover, S. (2007) Avoiding clinical drift. *Psychotherapy Networker* Jan/Feb, 25–26.

Brown, P., Crawford, P. and Carter, R. (2006) *Evidence Based Health Communication*. Maidenhead: Open University Press.

Burke, B.L., Arkowitz, H. and Menchola, M. (2003) The efficacy of motivational interviewing: a meta-analysis of controlled clinical trials. *Journal of Consulting and Clinical Psychology* 71(5), 843–861.

Burnard, P. (1992) Developing confidence. *Nursing* 4(47), 9–10.

Burnard, P. (2003) Ordinary chat and therapeutic conversation: phatic communication and mental health nursing. *Journal of Psychiatric and Mental Health Nursing* 10, 678–682.

Burnard, P. and Morrison, P. (1988) Nurses' perceptions of their interpersonal skills: a descriptive study using Six Category Intervention Analysis. *Nurse Education Today* 8, 266–272.

Burnard, P. and Morrison, P. (1989) What is an interpersonally skilled person? A repertory grid account of professional nurses' views. *Nurse Education Today* 9, 384–391.

Burnard, P. and Morrison, P. (1991) Nurses' interpersonal skills: a study of nurses' perceptions. *Nurse Education Today* 11(1), 24–29.

Burns, I. and Bulman, C. (2000) *Reflective Practice in Nursing. The Growth of the Professional Practitioner*. Oxford, Blackwell Science.

Byrne, P. (2008) Mental health nursing in an ethnically diverse society, in: Morrissey, J., Keogh, B. and Doyle, L. (eds) *Psychiatric Mental Health Nursing, An Irish Perspective*. Dublin: Gill 7 Macmillan.

Callaghan, P. (2006) Culturally capable mental health nursing, in: Callaghan, P. and Waldock, H. (eds) *The Oxford Handbook of Mental Health Nursing*. Oxford: Oxford University Press, pp. 276–277.

Callaghan, P., Khalil, E. and Morres, I. (2010) A prospective evaluation of the transtheoretical model applied to exercise in young people. *International Journal of Nursing Studies* 47, 3–12.

Campinha-Bacote, J. (1999) A model and instrument for addressing culturally competent care. *Journal of Nursing Education Thorofare* 38(5), 203–207.

Campinha-Bacote, J. (2003) Many faces: addressing diversity in health care. Online *Journal of Issues in Nursing* 8(1), 1–8.

Canales, M.K. and Bowers, B. (2001) Expanding conceptualizations of culturally competent care. *Journal of Advanced Nursing* 36(1), 102–111.

Carson, J. and Gordon, L (2010) Recovery and well being: the new paradigms for mental health services. *British Journal of Well Being* 1(1), 18–21.

Carton, J.S., Kessler, E.A. and Pape, C.L. (1999) Nonverbal decoding skills and relationship well-being in adults. *Journal of Nonverbal Behavior* 23, 91–100.

Chirema, K.D. (2007) The use of reflective journals in the promotion of reflection and learning in post-registration nursing students. *Nurse Education Today* 27, 192–202.

Clark, D.M. (1989) Anxiety states: panic and generalized anxiety, in: K. Hawton, K., Salkovskis, P.M., Kirk, J. and Clark D.M. (eds) *Cognitive Behaviour Therapy for Psychiatric Problems: A Practical Guide*. Oxford: Oxford University Press, pp. 52–96.

Coleman, P.T., Goldman, J.S., Kugler, K. (2009) Emotional intractability: gender, anger, aggression and rumination in conflict. *International Journal of Conflict Management* 20(2), 113–131.

Cook, N., Phillips, B. and Sader, D. (2005) The Tidal Model as experienced by patients and nurses in a regional forensic unit. *Journal of Psychiatric and Mental Health Nursing* 12, 536–540.

Cooke, M. and Matarasso, B. (2005) Promoting reflection in mental health nursing practice: a case illustration using problem-based learning. *International Journal of Mental Health Nursing* 14, 243–248.

Cooper, L. (2009) Values-based mental health nursing practice, in: Callaghan, P., Playle, J. and Cooper, L. (eds) *Mental Health Nursing Skills*. Oxford: Oxford University Press, pp. 21–32.

Corcoran, J. and Pillai, V. (2007) A review of the research on solution-focussed therapy. *British Journal of Social Work* 39, 234–242.

Cotton, A. (2001) Private thoughts in public spheres: issues in reflection and reflective practice in nursing. *Journal of Advanced Nursing* 36(4), 512–519.

Craft, M. (2005) Reflective writing and nursing education. *Journal of Nursing Education* 44(2), 53–58.

Crawford, P., Brown, B. and Bonham, P. (2006) *Communication in Clinical Settings*. Cheltenham: Nelson Thornes, pp. 138–151.

Culley, L. (2001) Nursing, culture and competence, in: Culley, L. and Dyson, S. (eds) *Ethnicity and Nursing Practice*. Basingstoke: Palgrave.

Culley, L. and Dyson, S. (2001) Introduction: sociology, ethnicity and nursing practice, in: Culley, L. and Dyson, S. (eds) *Ethnicity and Nursing Practice*. Basingstoke: Palgrave.

Cully, S. (1992) Counselling skills: an integrative framework, in: Dryden, W. (ed.) *Integrative and Eclectic Therapy: a Handbook*. Buckingham: Open University Press.

Cushing, A. (2003) Interpreters in medical consultations, in: Tribe, R. and Raval, H. (eds) *Working with Interpreters in Mental Health*. London: Routledge.

De Shazer, S. and Berg, I.K. (1997) What works? Remarks on research aspects of solution-focussed brief therapy. *Journal of Family Therapy* 19, 121–124.

De Shazer, S., Berg, I.K., and Lipchik, E. et al. (1986) Brief therapy: focussed solution development. *Family Process* 25, 207–221.

Department of Health (2004) *Getting Over the Wall. How the NHS is Improving the Patient's Experience*. London: DH.

Department of Health (2004) *The Ten Essential Shared Capabilities: a framework for the whole of the mental health workforce*. London: DH.

Department of Health (2005) *Delivering Race Equality in Mental Health Care: An action plan for reform inside and outside services*. London: DH. Available at www.dh.gov.uk.

Department of Health (2006) *Best Practice Competencies and Capabilities for Pre-Registration Mental Health Nursing in England: The Chief Nursing Officer's Review of Mental Health Nursing*. London: DH.

Department of Health (2011) *No Health without Mental Health: a cross-government mental health outcomes strategy for people of all ages.* London: DH.

Desivilya, H.S. and Eizen, D. (2005) Conflict management in work teams: the role of social self-efficacy and group identification. *International Journal of Conflict Management* 16(2), 183–208.

Dewey, J. (1933) *How we Think: A restatement of the relation of reflective thinking of the educative process.* Boston: University Press.

Dickinson, A. (1982) *A Woman in Your own Right: Assertiveness and you.* London: Quartet Books.

Dolan, Y.M. (1991) *Resolving Sexual Abuse: Solution-focussed therapy and Eriksonian hypnosis for adult survivors.* New York: Norton.

Doucet, L., Jehn, K.A., Weldon, E., Chen, X.M. and Wang, Z.M. (2009) Cross-cultural differences in conflict management: an inductive study of Chinese and American managers. *International Journal of Conflict Management* 20(4), 355–376.

Durgahee, T. (1998) Facilitating reflection: from a sage on stage to a guide on the side. *Nurse Education Today* 18, 158–164.

Egan, G. (2010) *The Skilled Helper*, 9th edn. Pacific Grove, CA: Brookes/Cole.

Evans, K. (2001) Expectations of newly qualified nurses. *Nursing Standard* 15(41), 33–38.

Eyton, A., Bischoff, A., Rrustemi et al. (2002) Screening of mental disorders in asylum-seekers from Kosovo. *Australian and New Zealand Journal of Psychiatry* 36, 499–503.

Fairbairn, C. and Cooper, P. (1989) Eating disorders in the UK, in: Hawton, P.M., Salkovskis, J., Kirk, J. and Clark, D.M. (eds) *Cognitive Behaviour Therapy for Psychiatric Problems: A practical guide.* Oxford: Oxford University Press, pp. 277–314.

Farrell, G.A. (2001) From tall poppies to squashed weeds: why don't nurses pull together more? *Journal of Advanced Nursing* 35(1), 26–33.

Felton, A. and Stickley, T. (2004) Pedagogy, power and service user involvement. *Journal of Psychiatric and Mental Health Nursing* 11, 89–98.

Fennell, M. (1989) Depression, in: Hawton, K., Salkovskis, P.M., Kirk, J. and Clark, D.M. (eds) *Cognitive Behaviour Therapy for Psychiatric Problems: A practical guide.* Oxford: Oxford University Press, pp. 169–234.

Fernando, S. (2003) Culture and ethnicity, in: Hannigan, B. and Coffee, M. (eds) *The Handbook of Community Mental Health Nursing.* London: Routledge.

Flanagan, J. (1954) The critical incident technique. *Psychological Bulletin* 51(4), 327–358.

Fleuren, M., Vander Meulen, M., Grol, R., DeHaan, M. and Wijkel, D. (1998) Does the care given by general practitioners and midwives to patients with (imminent) miscarriage meet the wishes and expectations of the patients? *International Journal for Quality in Health Care* 10, 213–220.

Fowler, J. (1995) Nurses' perceptions of the elements of good supervision. *Nursing Times* 91(22), 33–37.

Freshwater, D. (2003) *Counselling Skills for Nurses, Midwives and Health Visitors.* Maidenhead: Open University Press.

Fulford, K.W.M. (2004) Ten principles of values-based medicine, in: Radden, J. (ed.) *The Philosophy of Psychiatry: A companion.* New York: Oxford University Press, pp. 205–236.

Fulton, Y. (1997) Nurses' view on empowerment: a critical social theory perspective. *Journal of Advanced Nursing* 26(3), 529–536.

Gelder, M.G. (1989) Foreword, in: Hawton, K., Salkovskis, P.M., Kirk, J. and Clark, D.M. (eds) *Cognitive Behaviour Therapy for Psychiatric Problems: A practical guide.* Oxford: Oxford University Press.

Gellis, Z.D. and Kenaley, B. (2008) Problem-solving therapy for depression in adults: a systematic review. *Research in Social Work Practice* 18(2), 117–131.

Ghaye, T. and and Lillyman, S. (1997) *Learning Journals and Critical Incidents: Reflective practice for health care professionals.* Salisbury: Quay Books.

Gibbs, G. (1988) *Learning by Doing: A guide to teaching and learning methods.* Oxford: Further Education Unit, Oxford Brookes University.

Giger, J.N. and Davidhizar, R.E. (1999) *Transcultural Nursing: Assessment and intervention,* 3rd edn. St Louis: Mosby.

Gilburt, H., Rose, D. and Slade, M. (2008) The importance of relationships in mental health care: a qualitative study of service users' experiences of psychiatric hospital admission in the UK. Available at: http://www.Biomedcentral.com/1472–6963/8/92 (accessed 10 February 2010).

Gingerich, W.J. and Eisengart, S. (2000) Solution-focussed brief therapy: a review of the outcome research. *Family Process* 39, 477–498.

Glaze, J. (2001) Reflection as a transforming process: student advanced nurse practitioners' experience of developing reflective skills as part of an MSc programme. *Journal of Advanced Nursing* 37(3), 265–272.

Gleeson, M. and Higgins, A. (2009) Touch in mental health nursing: an exploratory study of nurses' views and perceptions. *Journal of Psychiatric and Mental Health Nursing* 16, 382–389.

Gopfert, M. (2002) Commentary on Iveson: solution-focussed brief therapy. *Advances in Psychiatric Treatment* 8, 149–157.

Gray, A. (1994) *An Introduction to the Therapeutic Frame.* London: Routledge, pp. 145–156.

Gray, J.A.M. (1997) *Evidence-based Health Care.* London: Churchill Livingstone.

Han, G. and Harms, P.D. (2010) Team identification, trust and conflict: a mediation model. *International Journal of Conflict Management* 21(1), 20–43.

Hannigan, B. (2001) A discussion in the strengths and weaknesses of 'reflection' in nursing practice and education. *Journal of Clinical Nursing* 10(2), 278–283.

Hargie, O. and Dickinson, D. (2004) *Skilled Interpersonal Communication: Research, theory and practice.* London: Routledge.

Heron, J. (1975) *Six Category Intervention Analysis.* Guildford: University of Surrey.

Heron, J. (1977) *Behavioural Analysis in Education and Training.* British Postgraduate Medical Federation, University of London and Guildford and University of Surrey, Surrey.

Heron, J. (1996) *Co-operative Inquiry: Research into the human condition.* London: Sage.

Heron, J. (1999) *The Complete Facilitator's Handbook.* London: Kogan Page.

Heron, J. (2001) *Helping the Client – A Creative Practical Guide,* 5th edn. London: Sage.

Hettema, J., Steele, J. and Miller, W.R. (2005) Motivational interviewing. *Annual Review of Clinical Psychology* 1, 91–111.

Hewitt, J., Coffey, M. and Rooney, G. (2009) Forming, sustaining and ending therapeutic interactions, in: Callaghan, P., Playle, J. and Cooper, L. (eds) *Mental Health Nursing Skills.* Oxford: Oxford University Press, pp. 63–73.

Hoffman, E. (1998). *Lost in Translation.* London: Vantage.

Hopkins, J.E., Loeb, S.J. and Fick, D.M. (2009) Beyond satisfaction, what service users expect of inpatient mental health care: a literature review. *Journal of Psychiatric and Mental Health Nursing* 16, 927–937.

Iley, K. and Nazroo, J. (2001) Ethnic inequalities in mental health, in: Culley, L. and Dyson, S. (eds) *Ethnicity and Nursing Practice.* Basingstoke: Palgrave.

Iveson, C. (2002) Solution-focussed brief therapy. *Advances in Psychiatric Treatment* 8, 149–157.

Jarvis, P. (1992) Reflective practice and nursing. *Nurse Education Today* 12, 174–181.

Jarvis, P., Holford, J. and Griffin, C. (2003) *The Theory and Practice of Learning,* 2nd edn. London: Kogan Page.

Jensen, J. (2000) Portrait of a person with schizophrenia. *Journal of Psychosocial Nursing and Mental Health Services* 29, 46–50.

Johns, C. (2000) *Becoming a Reflective Practitioner*. London: Blackwell Science.

Jones, C., Cormac, I., Mota, J. and Campbell, C. (2000) Cognitive behaviour therapy for schizophrenia (Cochrane Review), in: *The Cochrane Library*, Issue 2. Oxford: Update Software.

Kai, J. and Crosland, A. (2001) People with enduring mental health problems describe the importance of communication, continuity of care and stigma. *British Journal of General Practice* 51, 730–736.

Kamile, K., Kadriye, B., Ozen, K. et al. (2006) The effects of locus of control, communication skills and social support on assertiveness in female nursing students. *Social Behaviour and Personality* 32, 27–40.

Kemp, R., Hayward, P., Applewhaite, G., Everitt, B. and David, A. (1996) Compliance therapy in psychotic patients: randomised controlled trial. *British Medical Journal* 312: 345–349.

Kilkus, S.P. (1993) Assertiveness among professional nurses. *Journal of Advanced Nursing* 18, 1324–1330.

Kim, J.S. (2008) Examining the effectiveness of solution-focussed brief therapy: a meta-analysis. *Research on Social Work Practice* 18(2), 107–116.

Kim, J.S. and Franklin, C. (2009) Solution-focussed brief therapy in schools: a review of the outcome literature. *Children and Youth Services Review* 464–470.

Kitwood, T. and Bredin, K. (1992) A new approach to the evaluation of dementia care. *Journal of Advances in Health and Nursing Care* 1, 41–60.

Koivisto, K., Janhonen, S. and Vaisanen, L. (2004) Patients' experiences of being helped in an inpatient setting. *Journal of Psychiatric Mental Health Nursing* 11, 268–275.

Lago, C. and Thompson, J. (1996) *Race, Culture and Counselling*. Buckingham: Open University Press.

Larijani, T.T., Aghajani, M., Baheiraei, A. and Neiestanak, N.S. (2010) Relation of assertiveness and anxiety among Iranian university students. *Journal of Psychiatric and Mental Health Nursing* 17, 893–899.

Layard, R. (2005) *Happiness: Lessons from a new science*. London: Penguin.

Lee, L.J., Batal, H.A., Masselli, J.H. and Kutner, J.S. (2002) Effect of Spanish interpretation method on patient satisfaction in an urban walk-in clinic. *Journal of General Internal Medicine* 17, 641–646.

Leininger, M. (1978) *Transcultural Nursing: Concepts, theories and practices*. New York: Wiley & Sons.

Leininger, M. (1995) *Culture Care Diversity and Universality: A theory of nursing*. New York: National League for Nursing.

Lindberg, J.B., Hunter, M.L. and Kruszewski, A.Z. (1983) *Introduction to Person-centered Nursing*. Philadelphia, PA: Lippincott.

Liu, J., Fu, P. and Liu, S. (2009) Conflicts in top management teams and team/firm outcomes: the moderating effects of conflict-handling approaches. *International Journal of Conflict Management* 20(3), 228–250.

Lyubomirsky, S. (2008) *The How of Happiness: A scientific approach to getting the life you want*. New York: Penguin Press.

Mac Kay, R., Hughes, J. and Carver, E. (1990) *Empathy in the Helping Relationship*. New York: Springer Publishing.

Madhok, R., Bhopal, R.S., Ramaiah, R.S. (1992) Quality of hospital service: a study comparing Asian and non-Asian patients in Middlesbrough. *Journal of Public Health Medicine* 14, 271–279.

Maneesakorn, S., Robson, D., Gournay, K. and Gray, R. (2007) An RCT of adherence therapy for people with schizophrenia in Chiang Mai, Thailand. *Journal of Clinical Nursing* 16, 1302–1312.

Mann, S. and Cowburn, J. (2005) Emotional labour and stress within mental health nursing. *Journal of Psychiatric and Mental Health Nursing* 12, 152–162.

Mantzoukas, S. and Jasper, M.A. (2004) Reflective practice and daily ward reality: a covert power game. *Journal of Clinical Nursing* 13, 925–933.

Maslow, A. (1970) *Motivation and Personality*, 2nd edn. New York: Harper and Row.

McCabe, C. and Timmins, F. (2006) *Communication Skills for Nursing Practice*. London: Palgrave Macmillan.

McCartan, P.J. and Hargie, O.D. (2004) Assertiveness and caring: are they compatible? *Journal of Clinical Nursing* 13, 707–713.

McGrath, D. and Higgins, A. (2006) Implementing and evaluating reflective practice group session. *Nurse Education in Practice* 6, 175–181.

Meichenbaum, D. (1997) Cognitive behaviour therapy, in: Baum, A., Newman, S., Weinman, J., West, R. and McManus, C. (eds) *Cambridge Handbook of Psychology, Health and Medicine*. Cambridge: Cambridge University Press, pp. 200–203.

Miller, W.R. and Rollnick, S. (2002) *Motivational Interviewing: Preparing people for change, Vol. 2*. New York: Guilford.

Molassiotis, A., Callaghan, P., Twinn, S.F., Lam, S.W., Chung, W.Y. and Li, C.K. (2002) A pilot study of the effects of cognitive-behavioural group therapy and peer support/counselling in decreasing psychological distress and improving quality of life in Chinese symptomatic HIV patients. *AIDS Patient Care and STDs* 16(2), 83–96.

Mooney, M. (2007) Professional socialization: the key to survival as a newly qualified nurse. *International Journal of Nursing Practice* 13, 75–80.

Moos, R.H. (1997) *Evaluating Treatment Environments: The quality of psychiatric and substance abuse programs*. New Brunswick, NJ: Transaction.

Morrissey, J. (2009) Interpersonal communication – Heron's Six Category Intervention Analysis, in: Callaghan, P., Playle, J. and Cooper, L. (eds) *Mental Health Nursing Skills*. Oxford: Oxford University Press, pp. 56–62.

Morse, J.M., Bottorff, J., Anderson, G., O'Brien, B. and Solberg, S. (1992) Beyond empathy: expanding expressions of caring. *Journal of Advanced Nursing* 17, 809–821.

Morse, J.M., Miles, M., Clarke, D. and Doberneck, B. (1994) Sensing patient needs: exploring concepts of nursing insight and receptivity used in nursing assessment. *Scholarly Inquiry for Nursing Practice* 8, 233–260.

Moyle, W. (2003) Nurse–patient relationship: a dichotomy of expectations. *International Journal of Mental Health Nursing* 12, 103–109.

Myles, P. and Richards, D. (2006) Clinical skills for primary care mental health practice, in: *Primary Care Mental Health CD-Rom 3*. Centre for Clinical and Academic Workforce Innovation, University of Lincoln.

Mynors-Wallace, L. and Lau, M.E. (2010) Problem solving as a low intensity intervention, in: Bennett-Levy et al. (eds) *Oxford Guide to Low Intensity CBT Interventions*. Oxford: Oxford University Press, pp. 151–158.

Nair, N. (2008) Towards understanding the role of emotions in conflict: a review and future directions. *International Journal of Conflict Management* 19(4), 359–381.

Narayanasamy, A. (2003) Transcultural nursing: how do nurses respond to cultural needs? *British Journal of Nursing* 12(3), 185–195.

NHS Institute for Innovation and Improvement (2008) *Managing Conflict*. Accessed from http://www.institute.nhs.uk/quality_and_service_improvement_tools/quality_and_service_improvement_tools/human_dimensions_-_managing_conflict.html (accessed 24 May 2010).

NHS III Quality and Service Improvement Tools, Managing Conflict, London: Department of Health.

NHS Modernisation Agency (2003) *Essence of Care, Guidance and New Communications Benchmarks*. London: Department of Health.

Nicholl, H. and Higgins, A. (2004) Reflection in preregistration nursing curricula. *Journal of Advanced Nursing* 46(6), 578–585.

Nursing and Midwifery Council (2002) *Code of Professional Conduct*. London: NMC.

Nursing and Midwifery Council (2008) *The Code: Standards of conduct, performance and ethics for nurses and midwives*. London: NMC.

O'Carroll, M. (2006) Cognitive behaviour therapy, in: Callaghan, P. and Waldock, H. (eds) *The Oxford Handbook of Mental Health Nursing*. Oxford: Oxford University Press, p. 144.

O'Connell, B. (1998) *Solution-focussed Therapy*. London: Sage.

Papadopolous, I. (2001) Antiracism, multi-culturalism and the third way, in: Baxter, C. (ed.) *Managing Diversity and Inequality in Health Care*. Edinburgh: Bailliere.

Pardey, D. (2007) *Introducing Leadership*. Oxford: Butterworth Heineman, pp. 159–170.

Peplau, H. (1952) *Interpersonal Relations in Nursing*. New York: Putnam.

Peplau, H. (1997) Peplau's Theory of Interpersonal Relations. *Nursing Science Quarterly* 10(4), 162–167.

Phillips, P. and Callaghan, P. (2009) Working with people with substance misuse problems, in: Callaghan, P., Playle, J. and Cooper, L. (eds) *Mental Health Nursing Skills*. Oxford: Oxford University Press, pp. 203–212.

Platzer, H., Blake, D. and Ashford, D. (2000) An evaluation of process and outcomes from learning through reflective practice groups on a post-registration nursing course. *Journal of Advanced Nursing* 31(3), 689–695.

Pondy, L.R. (1966) A systems theory of organizational conflict. *Academy of Management Journal* 9(3), 246–256.

Poroch, D. and McIntosh, W. (1995) Barriers to assertive skills in nurses. *Australian and New Zealand Journal of Mental Health Nursing* 4, 113–123.

Price, J.R. and Cooper, J. (2000) Cognitive behaviour therapy for adults with chronic fatigue syndrome (Cochrane review), in: *The Cochrane Library*, Issue 2. Oxford: Update Software.

Price, K.M. and Cortis, J.D. (2000) The way forward for transcultural nursing. *Nurse Education Today* 20, 233–243.

Prochaska, J.O. and Marcus, B.H. (1994) the transtheoretical model: applications to exercise, in: Dishman, R. (ed.) *Advances in Exercise Adherence. Volume 2*. Illinois: Human Kinetic Press.

Punwar, J. and Peloquin, M. (2000) *Occupational Therapy: Principles and practice*. Philadelphia: Lippincott, p. 285.

Rack, P. (1982) *Race, Culture and Mental Disorder*. London: Tavistock Publications.

Rakos, R.F. (2003) Asserting and confronting, in: Hargie, O.D.W. (ed.) *The Handbook of Communication Skills*, 2nd edn. London: Routledge.

Raval, H. (2003) *Working with Interpreters in Mental Health*. London: Routledge.

Razban, M. (2003). An interpreter's perspective, in: Tribe, R. and Raval, H. (eds) *Working with Interpreters in Mental Health*. London: Routledge.

Repper, J. (2000) Adjusting the focus of mental health nursing: Incorporating service users' experiences of recovery. *Journal of Mental Health* 9(6), 575–587.

Reynolds, W.J. and Scott, B. (1999) Empathy: a crucial component of the helping relationship. *Journal of Psychiatric Mental Health Nursing* 6(5), 363–370.

Reynolds, W.J. and Scott, B. (2000) Do nurses and other professional helpers normally display much empathy? *Journal of Advanced Nursing* 31(1), 226–234.

Richards, D. (2010) Behavioural activation, in: Bennett-Levy J. et al (eds) *Oxford Guide to Low Intensity CBT Interventions*. Oxford: Oxford University Press, pp. 141–150.

Richards, D. and Whyte, M. (2009) *Reach Out: National Programme Student Materials to Support the Delivery of Training for Psychological Well Being Practitioners Delivering Low Intensity Interventions.* London: Rethink.

Rogers, C. (1961) *On Becoming a Person.* London: Constable.

Rogers, C. (1990) *A Way of Being.* Boston: Houghton Mifflin.

Rolfe, G., Jasper, M. and Freshwater, D. (2010) *Critical Reflection in Practice, Generating Knowledge for Care,* 2nd edn. London: Palgrave Macmillan.

Rosenberg, M. (1965) *Society and the Adolescent Self-image.* Princeton, NJ: Princeton University Press.

Roth, A. and Fonagy, P. (2005) *What Works for Whom? A Critical Review of Psychotherapy Research,* 2nd edn. New York: Guilford Press.

Rowan, J. (2001) *Ordinary Ecstasy: Dialectics of humanistic psychology,* 3rd edn. London: Routledge.

Sackett, D., Rosenburg, W., Gray, J.A.M., Haynes, B. and Richardson, W.S. (1996) Evidence-based medicine: what it is and what it is not. *British Medical Journal* 312, 71–72.

Sainsbury Centre for Mental Health (1998) *Acute Problems: A survey of the quality of care in acute psychiatric wards.* London: Sainsbury Centre for Mental Health.

Salkovskis, P.M. and Kirk, J. (1989) Obsessional disorders, in: Hawton, K., Salkovskis, P.M., Kirk, J. and Clark, D.M. (eds) *Cognitive Behaviour Therapy for Psychiatric Problems: A practical guide.* Oxford: Oxford University Press, pp. 129–168.

Schön, D. (1983) *The Reflective Practitioner: How professionals think in action.* London: HarperCollins.

Schön, D. (1987) *Educating the Reflective Practitioner.* San Francisco, CA: Jossey-Bass.

Scottish Executive (Government) (2006) *Rights, Relationships and Recovery: The Report of the National Review of Mental Health Nursing in Scotland.* Edinburgh: Scottish Executive.

Seedhouse, D. (2005) *Values-based Decision Making for the Caring Profession.* Chichester: Wiley.

Seligman, M., Rashid, T. and Parks, A. (2006) Positive psychology. *American Psychologist* 61(8), 774–788.

Sensky, T., Turkington, D., Kingdon, D. et al. (2000) A randomized controlled trial of cognitive-behavioural therapy for persistent symptoms in schizophrenia resistant to medication. *Archives of General Psychiatry* 57, 165–172.

Shepherd, G., Boardman, J. and Slade, M. (2009) *Ten Top Tips for Recovery-oriented Practice.* London: Sainsbury Centre for Mental Health.

Shih, H.A. and Susantoi, E. (2010) Conflict management styles, emotional intelligence, and job performance in public organisations. *International Journal of Conflict Management* 21(2), 147–168.

Somerville, D. and Keeling, J. (2004) A practical approach to promote reflective practice within nursing. *Nursing Times* 100(12), 42–45.

Speakman, J. and Ryals, L. (2010) A re-evaluation of conflict theory for the management of multiple, simultaneous conflict episodes. *International Journal of Conflict Management* 21(2), 186–201.

Spence, J. (1991) *The Search for Modern China.* New York: Norton.

Squier, R. (1990) A model of empathic understanding and adherence to treatment regimes in practitioner–patient relationships. *Social Science Medicine* 30, 325–339.

Stevenson, C. (2008) Therapeutic communication in mental health nursing, in: Morrissey, J., Keogh, B. and Doyle, L. (eds) *Psychiatric/Mental Health Nursing: An Irish perspective.* Dublin: Gill & Macmillan.

Stickley, T. and Stacey, G. (2009) Caring: the essence of mental health nursing, in: Callaghan, P., Playle, J. and Cooper, L. (eds) *Mental Health Nursing Skills.* Oxford: Oxford University Press.

Sully, P. and Dallas, J. (2005) *Essential Communication Skills for Nursing*. London: Elsevier Mosby.

Sundstrom, S.M. (1993) Single session psychotherapy for depression: is it better to be problem focussed or solution focussed? Unpublished doctoral dissertation, Iowa State University, Ames.

Thomas, J.L., Bliese, P.D. and Jex, S.M. (2005) Interpersonal conflict and organisational commitment: examining two levels of supervisory support as multi-level moderators. *Journal of Applied Social Psychology* 35(11), 2375–2398.

Timmins, F. and McCabe, C. (2005) Nurses' and midwives' assertive behavior in the workplace. *Journal of Advanced Nursing* 51(1), 38–45.

Tribe, R. (1998) If two is company is three a crowd/group? A longitudinal account of a support and clinical supervision group for interpreters. *Group Work Journal* 11, 139–152.

Tribe, R. (2004) Working with interpreters in legal and forensic settings, in: Barrett, K. and George, B. (eds) *Race, Culture, Psychology and the Law*. New York: Sage.

Tribe, R. and Morrissey, J. (2003) The refugee context and the role of interpreters, in Tribe, R. and Raval, H. (eds) *Working with Interpreters in Mental Health*. London: Routledge.

Tribe, R. and Morrissey, J. (2004) Good practice issues in working with interpreters in mental health. *Intervention* 2(2), 129–142.

University of Wisconsin Office of Human Resource Development (2006) *Conflict Resolution*. Accessed at http://www.ohrd.wisc.edu/onlinetraining/resolution/stepsoverview.

Warren, B.J. (2003) Cultural competence in psychiatric nursing, in: Keltner, A., Schwelke, T. and Bostrom, R. (eds) *Psychiatric Nursing*, 4th edn. New York: Mosby.

Watson, W.H. (1975) The meaning of touch: geriatric nursing. *Journal of Communication* 23, 104–112.

Webne-Behrman, H. (1998) *The Practice of Facilitation: Managing group processes and solving problems*. Wisconsin: Greenwood Publishing.

Williams, C. (1992) Where has all the empathy gone? *Professional Nurse* 8, 134.

Williams, C. and Chellingsworth, M. (2010) *CBT: A clinician's guide to using the Five Areas approach*. London: Hodder Arnold.

Wong, F.K.Y., Lok, Y., Wong, M., Tse, H., Kan, E. and Kember, D. (1997) An action research study into the development of nurses as reflective practitioners. *Journal of Nursing Education* 36, 476–481.

Woodbridge, K. and Fulford, K.W.M. (2004) Good practice? Values-based practice in mental health. *Mental Health Practice* 7(2), 30–34.

Yoshioka, M. (2000) Substantive differences in the assertiveness of low-income African American, Hispanic and Caucasian women. *Journal of Psychology* 134, 243–259.

Zarankin, T. (2007) A new look at conflict styles: goal orientation and outcome preferences. *International Journal of Conflict Management* 19(2), 167–184.

Index